Clinical Purification

A Complete Treatment and Reference Manual

An Ancestral Approach to Preventing and Reversing
the Disease Process, Validated by Modern Science

Gina L. Nick, Ph.D., N.D.

Published by:

Longevity Through Prevention, Inc.

PO Box 627

Brookfield, WI 53008

(866) 587-4622

e-mail : publisher@ltponline.com

(for orders and customer service inquiries)

Cover Design, Book Layout & Design by
Raymond Bonavida – Drawbridge Graphic Design Services

Illustrations by Raymond Bonavida and Amy Friemoth

Select Herb photographs copyright Steven Foster

Library of Congress Control Number: 2001094952

ISBN 0-9712118-0-9

LTP

PRINTED IN THE U.S.A.

NOTE TO THE READER

This book is meant to be a source of information for those interested in learning about how the Clinical Purification™ process can help cleanse and balance the body and promote better health. Whenever one speaks about health and disease, it is well known that biochemical individuality, lifestyle, diet, psychological state and spiritual maturity will affect a person's response to most therapeutic modalities. The author's intent is to share her experience and research findings with healthcare professionals to help them become more informed about purification and detoxification processes and one's general state of health. This book is sold with the understanding that the author, Dr. Gina Nick, and the publisher, Longevity Through Prevention, Inc, disclaim any liability, loss, or risk, personal or otherwise, which is incurred as a consequence, directly or indirectly, of the use and application of the contents of this book. The information presented in this book is not intended to be a substitute for standard medical treatments as prescribed by a qualified healthcare practitioner.

Table of Contents

FOREWORD

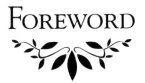

For several decades, many of the protocols of modern medicine have been established to treat the end result of the disease process. This strategy has hampered the progress of our fight against modern disease. A significant rise in the onset of degenerative diseases currently plagues our society and there is certainly no shortage of theories on causative factors. It has not been until recently however, that emphasis has been placed on the prevention of disease through dietary and lifestyle changes.

Modern health care practitioners are faced with making decisions daily about the best way to assist their patients in treating diseases. For thousands of years we, as a species, have recognized that certain foods–real unaltered foods– provide a means to both repair the damages of ill health and prevent diseases from occurring. It is this key foundational understanding that Dr. Nick presents in this book. Her passion for communicating this "ancestral" wisdom undoubtedly will spark your own fire of passion in the battle against disease.

Our modern world is an extremely toxic place in which to live. The daily onslaught to our bodies from air pollution, water pollution, pesticides, herbicides, household cleansers, PCB's, dioxins and other chemicals places an overwhelming burden on our innate detoxification systems. The slow evolution of these systems over thousands of years has not kept pace with the demands placed on them today. In addition, the lack of nutrition available from real foods in the modern diet causes our bodies to begin to fail from the resulting toxic overload. The average American annually consumes 64 dozen donuts, over 50 gallons of soda pop, nearly 200 pounds of refined sugars, and over 4 pounds of food additives and preservatives. These are not the foods of our ancestors from which the species grew and survived. The need for regular detoxification assistance in our lives has become a reality. Dr. Nick shares this vision in the pages to follow with a modern scientific validation of these ancestral principles.

The theories presented in this book will certainly stimulate discussion and gain the attention of practitioners of medical science. Hopefully, it will encourage those of us charged with the responsibility of helping others to initiate long-term preventative studies to enhance the process even further. The framework and details for solving the dilemma we face are presented here: Living in today's world and surviving in optimal health facing the challenges of our own toxic environments.

The battle looms large before each of us. I am honored to share in the vision brought forth in these pages by Dr. Nick, that we have always had an answer to our problem through the use of real whole foods. Let these pages inspire you as they have me to carry the wisdom of our ancestors forward to your own life and those whom you serve. The health of each of us, and ultimately planet earth, is at stake. If indeed we are to survive, we need our combined effort to face these challenges.

David Minzel, PhD, CNC
Shoreline, Washington

PREFACE

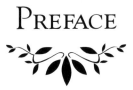

As a Naturopathic Physician, I have been exposed to a variety of dynamic healing protocols that include the use of nutrition, homeopathy, exercise, herbs, acupuncture, manipulation, pharmaceutical agents, emotional clearing, hydrotherapy, and surgery. By far, the most intriguing healing modality that I have encountered, both as a patient and as a physician, is the dynamic process of cleansing toxins from one's system primarily through the use of whole foods and herbs; the process of Clinical Purification™. I believe that Clinical Purification™ is a key to the prevention and treatment of the majority of health-related challenges that we face today, whether the cause of the challenge is spiritual, mental, emotional or physical.

This book embodies the results of nine years of exploration, as a researcher and as a clinician, into the area of detoxification. The result of this research serves to scientifically define, validate, and teach the complete process of cleansing toxins from one's body, with the use of whole unadulterated foods and herbs. I wrote this book because I saw the need for a well-documented source of information that teaches the countless benefits of a structured purification program that works. By discovering the interconnections between toxins, lifestyle, the foods that we eat and health, I hope that this work serves to convey to you the innumerable benefits of learning, practicing and teaching the Clinical Purification™ process.

I believe that the practice of effectively and safely cleansing toxins from one's body is a key to health and longevity, a secret so to speak, that has been well kept. Moreover, aside from the power of Love, there are few notions about healing the body that I know of that can have such a profound positive impact on one's journey through life.

In Health and Light.

ACKNOWLEDGEMENTS

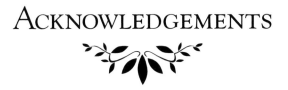

"If I have seen further than others, it is by standing upon the shoulders of giants."
—Newton

My gratitude to:

The many great teachers, both formal and informal, that have guided me throughout my educational career. A special thanks to the educators associated with Southwest College of Naturopathic Medicine and Health Sciences.

Dr. Michael Cronin, whose commitment to formally educating natural healers coupled with his genuine passion for naturopathic medicine inspired me to seek out an education at the college he founded, SCNM.

The SP family, starting with Dr. Royal Lee and continuing on with Charles DuBois, who, through their work and dedication to nutrition and the proper use of supplements, continue to fuel my vision of educating the world about the truths that I have been fortunate enough to discover concerning nutrition and healing.

Joseph Leonard, M.S., for providing me with great research and editorial assistance, and for honoring me with his presence in my professional life.

Dr. David and Judith Minzel, who, in the blink of an eye, carried me to a higher place professionally, personally and spiritually.

Brian and Anna Maria Clement and the staff at the Hippocrates Health Institute and the staff at the Optimum Health Institute for dedicating their lives to lovingly educating people on the inherent power and life-giving energy contained within whole, unadulterated foods, and for inspiring us all to take control of our own health and realize that disease is not a death sentence but merely a wake up call.

My parents, for paving a well lit road infused with wisdom, kindness and love, from which I am most proud to walk (and sometimes sprint) down, and my sister Fedora, who continually protects me from harm's way.

And most importantly, my husband, soul mate and very best friend Noah whose love and trust in me and my knowledge about health has inspired me to seek out the truth, always.

PART 1

TOXINS

"Disease is the retribution of outraged Nature."
—Ballou

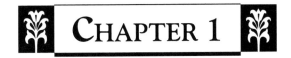

CHAPTER 1

THE HISTORY OF CLEANSING

"Time as he grows old teaches all things."
–Aeschylus

1

The History of Cleansing

At the turn of the sixth century, the ancient Greeks developed the Doctrine of Humors ascribing the notion that the body contained four humors – yellow bile, black bile, phlegm, and blood – that must remain in a state of equilibrium to maintain health. This doctrine formed the basis of ancient medical pathology. For centuries following the development of the Doctrine of Humors, the treatment of illness focused on balancing the humors using diet, bloodletting, cupping, enemas, vomiting, purging, and other purification techniques. Without exception, every culture used several of these techniques to cleanse and balance an ailing body. **Bloodletting** was a common cleansing practice in which ancient physicians would open a vein or use leeches to divert blood away from the symptomatic area. **Cupping** involved burning a piece of hemp in a cup until it burned out, then placing the cup over a cut. As it cooled, the vacuum in the cup suctioned blood out of the body. **Enemas** were used as a cleansing procedure and standard first line of care for nearly every illness, injury, or health problem.[40] Enemas, cupping, and leeches are still used today, although to a lesser extent by physicians and other healthcare practitioners.

Ancient physicians used **cathartics** (purgatives), substances that cause an active movement of the bowels, to cleanse the digestive tract. Psyllium seeds and husks were a popular cathartic that healthcare practitioners continue to use today. Most ancient civilizations also used **emetics** (substances that induce vomiting) to cleanse the body of harmful accumulations, increase the appetite, and promote digestion.

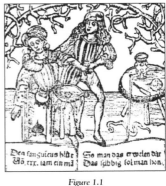

Figure 1.1
Woman being bled by a barber surgeon.
Brunschwig, Hieronymus. Published by
Johann (Reinhard) Grüninger, 1500. woodcut

Modern scientists have a better knowledge of gastrointestinal physiology and consequently have developed newer adaptations of these methods for aiding digestion using proper diet and herbal medicines.

Fasting (complete or partial abstinence from foods and liquids) was and still is an important means of purifying the body. Hippocrates and Maimonides, two of the most popular and effective healers of ancient cultures, were strong proponents of the use of fasting to detoxify the body and balance the humors.[40] **Massage, acupuncture, saunas,** and **baths** were also popular and effective detoxification methods used throughout history.

Today, modern medicine is controlled primarily by the practice of allopathic medicine, although an interest is reappearing for natural healthcare practices. The allopathic system of medicine defines health as the maintenance of a specific set of measurable lab values and vital signs. These measurable assessments of health include height, weight, electrolyte balance, blood pressure, temperature, visual acuity, respiratory rate, pulse rate, and auditory threshold. Cleansing or purification techniques are not primary constituents of allopathic practice. Rather, allopathic practitioners use drugs for the treatment of most health conditions, generally introducing more chemicals into a system that is already working under a toxic load. Patients with health challenges frequently are unable to effectively cleanse their systems of toxic loads, making them most vulnerable to the introduction of additional toxic elements, which must be cleared by the organ systems (in particular, the liver and kidneys). Informed healthcare practitioners have an effective and less dangerous tool kit to work with for treating even the most challenging cases. It involves the employment of select nutrient complexes and herbs in conjunction with a calorie restricted, nutrient dense diet aimed at clearing out toxins from the system. The complete process is known as Clinical Purification.™

Researchers are continually and consistently proving that Caloric Restriction, an important aspect to the Clinical Purification™ process retards aging in mammals and reduces the incidence of cancer.[12,38,46,47] Accordingly, appropriate changes can decrease the reparative and restorative requirements placed on the body, *allowing reactions to shift towards the elimination of stored toxins,* versus the elimination of exogenous and endogenous toxins that are introduced and produced when eating. It is important to insure that caloric restriction *does not introduce malnutrition.* This potential problem is overcome by using whole food and herbal complexes that supply the body with a concentrated mixture of essential nutrients and cofactors required for healthy cellular function.

A careful understanding of the nature of toxins and of the physiology behind the body's endogenous detoxification mechanisms is an important key to appreciating the elegant mechanisms of action of herbal remedies and whole food nutrient combinations and the complimentary effects of caloric restriction.

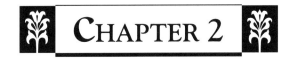

CHAPTER 2

INTERNAL TOXINS

*"What lies behind us and what lies before us
are tiny matters compared to what lies within us."*
—Emerson

2

INTERNAL TOXINS

The body produces and stores toxins of its own that require specific methods of detoxification to maintain homeostasis. Most internal toxins are produced as a by-product of cellular metabolic processes and include **dead and digested bacteria, hydrogen peroxide, cellular debris, and carbon dioxide**. Other sources of internal toxins include by-products produced by **an imbalance in tissue acid/alkali, ammonia, excess lactic acid**, and **endogenous free radical production. Microorganisms**, including bacteria, viruses, parasites, molds, yeast, and fungi, release metabolic products as they grow and multiply, many of which can be toxic and allergenic substances.

2.1   Acid / Alkaline Balance

Natural biochemical reactions in the body function to control acidity and alkalinity. These reactions produce waste products that, in excess, can be toxic to the system. A measure of whether a substance is acidic or alkaline with a scale that ranges from 0 to 14, is the **pH** factor. The neutral level value is seven, with all values below seven representing an acidic state and all values above seven representing an alkaline state.

Acid/alkali reactions in the body must occur at the proper speed and in the proper proportions or the body develops an acid/alkali imbalance. This imbalance produces toxins that cause damage. The gastrointestinal tract is an example of a physiologic system that is functionally dependent upon pH. In order to maintain homeostasis, the *mouth* should always be slightly alkaline, as salivary enzymes function in an alkaline environment; the *stomach* requires an acid environment for proper protein digestion; the *small intestine* contains pancreatic digestive enzymes that also require an alkaline environment to function properly; and the *large intestine* requires a slightly acidic environment to maintain proper bowel flora.[44]

In order to properly digest food, the liver and gallbladder must function synergistically with the varying pH environments within the intestinal tract. Interestingly, the liver is an embryonic outgrowth from the anterior part of the intestines. Liver cells secrete bile to the gallbladder which, when the gallbladder contracts, is forced into the bile duct and from there into the intestines if

Ph Values of Bodily and Other Substances

Gastric juices	1.2-3.0	**Acidic**
Lemon juice	2.2-2.4	
Vaginal fluid	3.5-4.5	
Urine	4.6-8.0	
Coffee	5.0	
Saliva	6.35-6.85	
Milk	6.6-6.9	
Pure water	7.0	
Blood	7.35-7.45	
Semen	7.2-7.6	
Cerebrospinal fluid	7.4	
Pancreatic juice	7.1-8.2	
Bile	7.6-8.6	
Lye	14.0	**Alkaline**

Figure 2.1
pH value of bodily and other fluids

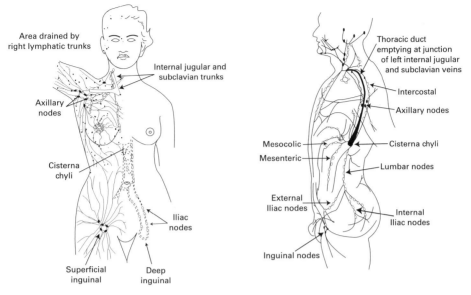

Figure 2.2
The lymphatic drainage system runs throughout the body.

food is present in the tract (the sphincter between the bile duct and the intestine remains closed until food enters). The bile plays a key role in the digestion of food as it is an alkaline substance that neutralizes the acidic chyme produced in the stomach, which in turn creates a favorable pH for pancreatic and intestinal enzymes to breakdown carbohydrates, protein and fat. Bile salts also function to emulsify fats, thereby facilitating fat product absorption. Figure 2.1 shows the wide variation in pH range of bodily fluids as well as ingested fluids that the body must work with to maintain homeostasis.

2.1.1 Connective Tissue and the Lymphatic Drainage System

Connective tissue relies on acid/alkaline balance to function properly. Also referred to as mesenchymal tissue, connective tissue consists of cells that support, connect, and anchor the structures of the body. A **lymphatic drainage system** exists in the connective tissue that essentially takes in toxic waste products and either releases them through the lymph system or stores them.

While the connective tissue is equipped to handle fluctuations in acid/alkaline balance, **excess exposure to acidic toxins causes mesenchymal acidosis that affects the magnesium and potassium balance of the cells, congests the lymphatic system, and disrupts calcium stores.**

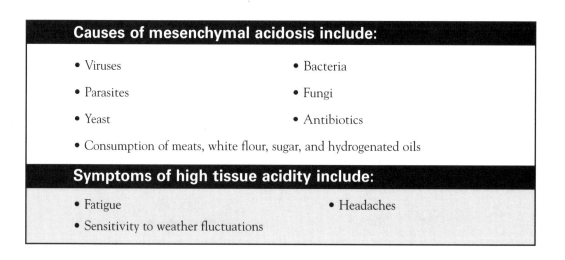

Causes of mesenchymal acidosis include:

- Viruses
- Parasites
- Yeast
- Consumption of meats, white flour, sugar, and hydrogenated oils
- Bacteria
- Fungi
- Antibiotics

Symptoms of high tissue acidity include:

- Fatigue
- Sensitivity to weather fluctuations
- Headaches

2.1.2 Respiration

Respiration is also intimately connected to acid/alkaline balance. Respiratory acidosis occurs when the body produces carbon dioxide at a faster rate than the lungs are able to expel it. As a result, carbonic acid levels increase in the blood and carbon dioxide and hydrogen ion levels elevate in the arteries, producing a toxic overload.

The body responds to this toxic overload by taking deeper, more rapid breaths to expel carbon dioxide. Under excessive conditions, hyperventilation occurs causing arterial concentrations of carbon dioxide and hydrogen ions to decrease, resulting in respiratory alkalosis, as carbon dioxide is eliminated more quickly than it is produced.

2.1.3 Blood pH

The pH of the blood is closely controlled by acid/alkaline buffer systems. Arterial, capillary, and venous blood is slightly alkaline, within a pH range of 7.30 to 7.45. If the pH of the blood exceeds this range, the system goes into **metabolic alkalosis**. Excessive vomiting, which rids the body of hydrochloric acid, and alkali therapy for peptic ulcers are a few causes of metabolic alkalosis which results in carbonate deposits in the bones, as the body pulls carbonate out of the blood in an attempt to lower the pH. **Metabolic acidosis** occurs when the blood pH falls below 7.3. A diabetic patient, for example, can be at risk for metabolic acidosis and coma because low levels of insulin cause abnormal glucose combustion, which in turn causes excessive acids to be produced in tissue metabolism. Hypoxia and severe exercise also produce metabolic acidosis, this time due to an excess production of lactic acid. Fasting and diarrhea cause metabolic acidosis as well. When the system is in metabolic acidosis for as little as two hours, bone dissolution occurs, whereby the body leaches carbonate out of the bone to help increase the pH of the blood. *The knowledgeable healthcare practitioner will be able to recognize subclinical and clinical signs of metabolic acidosis and alkalosis in order to properly prescribe whole food nutrient complexes and herbal medicines, an essential part of the Clinical Purification™ process, to aid the body in correcting the imbalance.*

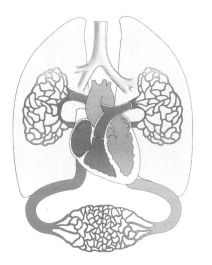 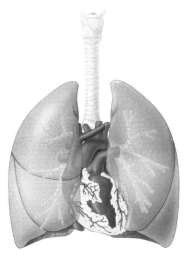

Circulatory System   The Lungs

Figure 2.3
The lungs and the circulatory system function synergistically to maintain acid/alkaline balance.

2.2 Endogenous Free Radicals

Normal biochemical processes in the body produce endogenous toxins or free radicals. **Free radicals** are chemically reactive pro-oxidants that are produced by the body and are necessary for life. They exist in limited numbers intracellularly and aid in defending the system against microbial attack. They also aid in activating enzyme reactions that are critical to hormone production. As some free radicals are a necessary part of normal metabolic reactions, the body supplies enzymes that control the free radicals, preventing them from causing damage in the body. However, if the free radicals are not kept under control, they become endogenous toxins, capable of damaging proteins, fats, and nucleic acids in the body. This can transduce a cascade of biochemical disruptions.

2.2.1 Emotional Trauma

Emotional trauma can also cause internal toxins to develop and affect health. Aristotle and Hippocrates documented the value of addressing emotional states when treating disease and assessing health. Psychological trauma and emotional, physical, and sexual abuse can all cause dysregulation of the central nervous system, resulting in toxic changes in brain chemistry and cells.

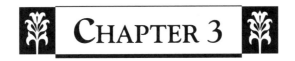

CHAPTER 3

EXTERNAL TOXINS

"America today stands poised on a pinnacle of wealth and power, yet we live in a land of vanishing beauty, of increasing ugliness, of shrinking open space, and of an over-all environment that is diminished daily by pollution and noise and blight."
—Udall

3

EXTERNAL TOXINS

The world's air, water, and food contain toxins that affect the health of all living things. Food contaminants, including pesticides, microorganisms and the toxins that they produce, additives, packaging materials, hormones, and heavy metals found in food are potentially toxic to the body. Gases and particulate matter in the air, including carbon monoxide, sulfur oxides, photochemical oxidants, hydrocarbons, asbestos, metals, and radio-nuclides are also toxic to the body and can potentially cause such health conditions as lung cancer, asthma, emphysema, and both acute and chronic respiratory and nonrespiratory conditions.[10,11,28] Chemicals and metals used in daily life cause environmental pollution that results in allergic sensitization and increased levels of IgE antibodies in the body.[35] **Children, the elderly, and fetuses are at an increased risk of developing toxic overload and sensitivity reactions to environmental pollutants. Specifically, fetuses are increasingly sensitive to lead, mercury, and polychlorinated biphenyls.[31,39]**

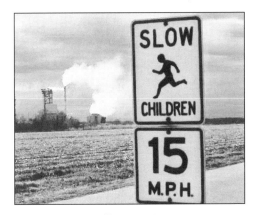

Figure 3.1
Children are at an increased risk for developing health challenges from exposure to environmental toxins.

Young children have an immature renal system, host detoxification process, and immune system, as well as a larger body surface area in relation to their weight.[31] The elderly patient often has an impaired drug detoxification system, an increase in fat tissue, and a loss of lean body mass, making him/her more susceptible to the adverse effects of environmental pollution. Females are reportedly also more susceptible than males to lead, benzene, and alcohol.[35]

3.1 Pesticides and Other Chemicals in Foods

Pesticides used on crops pose a major health threat to the body. Regulated in the U.S. by the Food and Drug Administration (FDA), the U.S. Department of Agriculture (USDA), and the Environmental Protection Agency (EPA), pesticides such as insecticides, herbicides, and fungicides can cause health challenges when organizations do not use them judiciously. Interestingly, 50% of all pesticides used are not detected by current testing methods for food contamination. Furthermore, U.S. manufacturers continue to produce pesticides that are banned, unregistered, or restricted by exporting them out of the U.S. Third World countries purchase the pesticides for crop maintenance and then sell these crops back to the U.S. for distribution. **DDT**, banned from the U.S. in 1973, still lingers in the fat cells of nearly 100% of the United States population, either as a residue of DDT or its metabolite DDE. It is present in the fatty tissue of fish, poultry, dairy products, and meat because it remains in our soil.[15]

3.1.1 Chlorinated Pesticides

Chlorinated pesticides primarily function in the body as neurotoxins. Chemicals like organochlorinated compounds (**OCCs**) interfere with axonal transmission. They disrupt the ion flux causing uncontrolled neuronal discharge. Chlorinated pesticides are known carcinogens and mutagens. Though they are generally classified as neurotoxins, chlorinated pesticides are also hemotoxic and immunotoxic. **Chlordane** is an example of a chlorinated pesticide with known risks to humans and wildlife that is still registered for use as a pesticide in the United States. This pesticide was primarily used to repel and kill termites by placing it in the soil under homes. It was also used on corn and other crops. By 1983, the EPA banned the production of chlordane for use under ground, due to concerns over its cancer causing effects, evidence of human exposure and build up in human fat cells, and its danger to wildlife. The latter danger became evident with the impact that this pesticide had on the Beluga whales in the St. Lawrence basin of Canada. Interestingly, there is no documented use of chlordane in the basin, yet it is found in the waters and sediments of this area. One hypothesis regarding its presence in this area is that the toxic chemical was carried into the seaway by winds blowing up from the southern U.S., where chlordane was once used heavily. The St. Lawrence basin drains a 500,000-square-mile area and any contaminant that rains down within its vast perimeter is, sooner or later, flushed into the area. This toxic chemical has been linked to the death of an indefinite number of Beluga whales in Canada.

Chlordane was still found on store shelves and used on the outside of homes to kill termites, but not underground, until April of 1988. The compound remains in the environment indefinitely, with evidence of its presence still found in food, air, water, and soil.   Due to its continued use on food crops and in houses to stop termites, almost every American has been exposed to small amounts of the chemical. The highest exposures to people today are from living in houses that were treated with chlordane for termites and from eating foods prepared from plants grown on chlordane-treated fields and the fat of meat and milk from animals that eat grass from chlordane-treated fields. At this time, chlordane has been found at 46 out of 1177 hazardous waste sites on the National Priorities List (NPL) in the United States.

More information regarding the impact of this toxic man-made substance on health, and on the risk of exposure, even today, to this substance may be found at the Agency for Toxic Substances and Disease Registry, Division of Toxicology, 1600 Clifton Road, E-29 Atlanta, Georgia 30333.

3.1.2 Organophosphates

Organophosphates are the primary class of pesticides used today. These pesticides phosphorylate acetylcholinesterase, resulting in the overstimulation of acetylcholine.

Long-term effects of organophosphate exposure include **axonal degeneration and myelin degeneration**, which cause conditions like multiple sclerosis. In addition, this class of pesticides decreases selenium levels in the brain and kidneys and stimulates the production of neurotoxin esterase causing peripheral neuropathies. Recently, a team of research scientists isolated a breakdown product of the popular pesticide methoxychlor that farmers readily use today on fruits and vegetables. The scientists found that HPTE, a by-product of this pesticide, interferes with levels of the hormone testosterone, affecting male fertility.[26] One of the members of the research team, Dr. Matthew Hardy, now cautions "protect yourself against exposure by eating organically grown fruits and vegetables."[26]

3.1.3 Polycyclic Aromatic Hydrocarbons

An additional group of toxic chemicals that we are exposed to is polycyclic aromatic hydrocarbons (**PAHs**). These chemicals are found in foods that have had contact with petroleum and coal tar products and are carcinogenic and mutagenic.[14] Scientists have made a direct association between PAHs and gastrointestinal cancer. It is documented that PAHs remain stored in the body fat, liver, adrenal glands, and ovaries.[14] All smoked foods and charbroiled foods contain some level of PAHs and a large percentage of seafood is contaminated with this chemical due to bioaccumulation from polluted water.

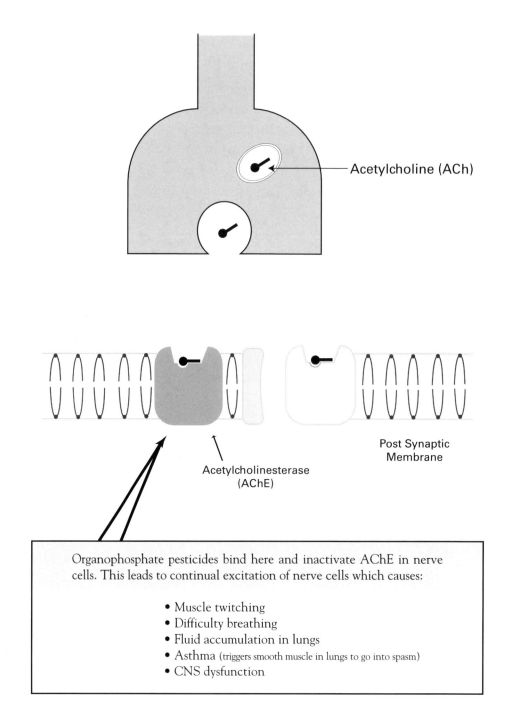

Acetylcholine (ACh)

Acetylcholinesterase
(AChE)

Post Synaptic
Membrane

Organophosphate pesticides bind here and inactivate AChE in nerve cells. This leads to continual excitation of nerve cells which causes:

- Muscle twitching
- Difficulty breathing
- Fluid accumulation in lungs
- Asthma (triggers smooth muscle in lungs to go into spasm)
- CNS dysfunction

Figure 3.2
Acetylcholine being released from a nerve cell. Organophosphates binding to acetylcholinesterase within nerves causes continuous excitation.

3.1.4 Polychlorinated Biphenyls, Metals, and Other Sources of Toxicity from the Environment

Other sources of toxicity from the external environment include industrial chemicals such as polychlorinated biphenyls (**PCBs**), metals such as lead and **mercury** (particularly as a result of mercury amalgam fillings used in dentistry), food packaging materials such as polyvinyl chloride and acrylonitrile, and food additives. Tetrachloroethylene, ethylbenzene, and benzene are toxic chemicals that were documented as being "everywhere present" in the air in a study completed by the EPA.[41] Dioxin is a toxic substance that is present as an emission from garbage incinerators and the pulp and paper industry. **The cancer risk from dioxin among individuals eating large amounts of dairy and fatty meat products is as high as 1 in 100,** a risk ten times larger than what has been reported previously. The U.S. Environmental Protection Agency reported that some of the general population has exposed itself to dioxin levels high enough to "pose serious health risks."[26]

Microorganisms and their metabolic products are another source of toxins in our food supply. Among the organisms most responsible for toxicity are *Staphylococcus aureus, Clostridium botulinum, Escherichia coli, Aspergillus spp.,* and *Claviceps pupurea.* These microorganisms cause a wide spectrum of health challenges. Their negative influence on health is seen in patients with a compromised biological terrain, where there is an increased growth of bacteria, yeast, fungi, and molds.

3.1.5 Cadmium

Cadmium is a naturally occurring element in the earth's crust. It is most often found in combination with other elements, such as oxygen (cadmium oxide), chlorine (cadmium chloride), and sulfur (cadmium sulfide). There are airborne and food sources of cadmium that place people at risk of increased exposure and resultant health hazards. The burning of fossil fuels, like coal or oil, and the incineration of municipal waste materials represent the largest airborne sources of cadmium.[2] The addition of phosphate fertilizers and sewage sludge increases cadmium levels in the soil, thus increasing the levels found in the food supply. Smoking is another source of cadmium, resulting in a 100% increase in the relative amount of cadmium found in smokers versus non-smokers. Cadmium

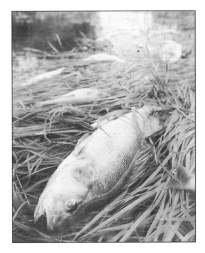

Figure 3.3
Cadmium bioaccumulates in the tissues of some fish as a result of pollution

is classified as a "pollutant of concern" to the EPA's Great Waters Program because of its potential to bioaccumulate, its toxicity to the environment and to the human body, and its persistence in the environment.[2]

Most cadmium used in the United States is a soft, bluish metal or grayish powder obtained as a by-product of the treatment of copper, lead, and iron ores. 35% of cadmium is used for metal plating, 25% for nickel-cadmium and other types of batteries, 20% for pigment dyes, 15% for plastic stabilizers, and 5% for other uses, including pesticides, alloys, and chemical reagents and/or intermediates.

Human and animal studies show an **increase in lung cancer** from exposure to inhaled cadmium.[2,6,13] **Chronic inhalation and oral exposure to cadmium has a cumulative toxic effect on the kidneys, causing proteinuria, increased frequency of kidney stone formation, and a decrease in glomerular filtration rate.**[2,6,42] There is evidence that cadmium causes prostate and kidney cancer in humans, and it has been shown to cause testicular cancer in animals.[13] It is a probable teratogen in humans. It may damage the testes and affect the female reproductive cycle. Specifically, cadmium accumulates in the ovaries, uterus, and testes, decreases the amount of growing follicles in the ovary, decreases the germinal epithelium, increases the stroma in testicles (increasing the risk of cancer), inhibits spermatozoa motility parameters *in vitro*, and decreases the weight of offspring.[32]

Signs and symptoms of long-term exposure to cadmium include:

- Anemia
- Loss of sense of smell
- Fatigue
- Yellow staining of teeth

Short-term health effects of exposure to cadmium include:

- A flu-like illness with chills, headache, aching, and/or fever
- Nausea
- Salivation
- Vomiting
- Cramps
- Diarrhea
- Rapid and severe lung damage with shortness of breath, chest pain, cough, and a buildup of fluid in the lungs
- Occasionally death

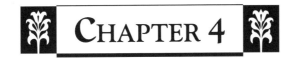

CHAPTER 4

HEALTH CHALLENGES
AND TOXICITY

*"It is more important to know what sort of patient has a
disease than to know what sort of disease has a patient."*
                                                    –Osler

4

HEALTH CHALLENGES
AND TOXICITY

Toxic exposure and compromised endogenous detoxification mechanisms cause a number of signs, symptoms, and associated health challenges. Common signs of toxicity syndromes include weight gain of unknown etiology, headaches, impaired resistance to bacterial and viral infections, arthritic pain, and lethargy.

Note that prenatal exposure to environmental toxins by the mother can cause adverse reactions that do not manifest until later in the child's life. For example, maternal exposure to mercury can cause low birth weight children and severe brain damage. Toluene exposure causes CNS dysfunction, developmental delay, craniofacial and limb abnormalities.[10,31,39] Exposure to polychlorinated biphenyls (PCBs) during pregnancy results in dark brown pigmentation, lower birth weight, and shorter gestation time.[35,39] Paternal exposure to toxins also presents risks to the fetus. Men who are exposed to vinyl chloride in the workplace cause an increased rate of spontaneous abortion in their wives.[35]

**Exposure to chemical substances also has
adverse effects on the developing child.**

Developmental toxicants cause:

- Low birth weight [35,39]
- Brain cancer [8,9,18,37]
- Metabolic and biologic dysfunction [35,36]
- Behavioral disorders and other birth defects [8,9,10,31,39]

4.1 Cancer

Environmental toxins (carcinogens) cause the majority of cancers seen today. Further, the probability of developing cancer due to toxic exposure increases exponentially when the body is deficient in nutrients specific for supporting endogenous detoxification mechanisms. Thus, supplying essential nutrient complexes that support the organ systems responsible for detoxification becomes a key factor in preventing the onset and/or progression of cancer. Positively, *there are multiple nutrients and herbs that have a documented chemo-protective action on the body.*[1,3,4,24,33,34,45] Environmental pollutants, prescription medications, and alcohol compromise the body's ability to detoxify. Specifically, **exposure to pesticides is linked to breast cancer,**[5] **leukocytopenia,**[35] **lymphatic and non-lymphatic leukemia, and soft tissue sarcoma. Exposure to industrial chemicals is linked to bladder cancer and exposure to cigarette smoke is linked to lung cancer.**[14] It is important to note that there is a wealth of scientifically valid, well-documented literature available on the health conditions associated with toxic exposure and damage to detoxification mechanisms, that are beyond the scope of this book.

The number of toxins that humans and animals are exposed to has increased multifold and continues to do so, compromising organs responsible for detoxification and causing serious health challenges. It is critical for physicians and healthcare practitioners to research this area of medicine further, so as to understand the mechanisms of action of pollutants, chemicals and heavy

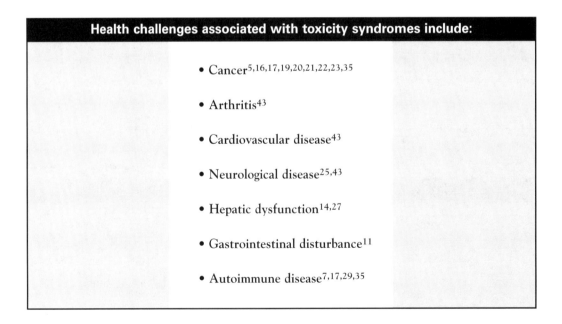

Health challenges associated with toxicity syndromes include:

- Cancer[5,16,17,19,20,21,22,23,35]

- Arthritis[43]

- Cardiovascular disease[43]

- Neurological disease[25,43]

- Hepatic dysfunction[14,27]

- Gastrointestinal disturbance[11]

- Autoimmune disease[7,17,29,35]

metals and their effects on human health. By doing so, practitioners and their patients will realize the many benefits of preventing and treating illness by preventing exposure to toxic elements and by providing long-term support for the detoxification organs in the body.

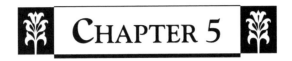

CHAPTER 5

ENDOGENOUS DETOXIFICATION MECHANISMS

"Medicine is not only a science; it is also an art. It does not consist of compounding pills and plasters; it deals with the very processes of life, which must be understood before they may be guided."
—Paracelsus

5
⇒≫)❈(≪⇐

ENDOGENOUS
DETOXIFICATION MECHANISMS

Multiple organ systems function to cleanse the body of exogenous and endogenous toxic substances including the liver, lungs, gastrointestinal tract and skin. Other routes of excretion include the kidneys, hair, nails, sweat, and breast milk. Some toxins actually target and damage the organs that are responsible for detoxification or block the routes of excretion, causing an excess accumulation of toxins in the body, resulting in intracellular damage and disease. Herbal medicines and whole food-based extracts contain nutritional and tertiary functional compounds that work synergistically to support and repair damage to these organ systems. Following is a brief overview of select organ systems involved in the process of detoxification.

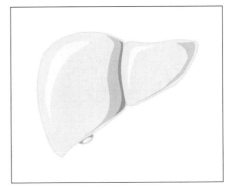

Figure 5.1
The Liver

5.1 The Liver

The liver plays a central role in the regulation of key metabolic functions in the body, including carbohydrate metabolism, fat metabolism, protein metabolism, storage of vitamins, and the removal of toxins and hormones from the body.

5.1.1 Biochemical Individuality and Liver Function

It is critical that practitioners and researchers realize the concept of biochemical individuality, particularly when it comes to the demonstrated variability between genders. Medical researchers often presume that, aside from the obvious morphological differences in reproductive organs between men and women, both genders react similarly to the metabolism of drugs. Consequently, research has focused primarily on the effects of drugs on liver detoxification enzymes in men, and not in women. However, phase I liver detoxification enzymes, such as CYP3A4, are induced by progesterone, implicating that liver function is affected by hormones, whose concentrations vary significantly between the sexes. With regard to the excretion of toxins via the liver, there can be no doubt that distinct influential differences in liver detoxification enzymes exist between men and women thereby affecting one's relative susceptibility and outcome to toxic exposure. The study of biochemical individuality warrants further attention, particularly as we look to the anatomical, physiological and biochemical effects of toxins on the body.

5.1.2 Removal or Excretion of Toxins

People today have an overwhelming exposure to external toxins that, compounded with the body's own toxin-producing capabilities, provides evidence for the need to support the functioning of detoxification organs in the body. Toxins increase the amount of free radicals in the body. Free radicals (pro-oxidants) are chemically reactive molecules, some of which are a necessary part of normal metabolic reactions. The body supplies enzymes that control free radicals, preventing them from causing tissue damage. However, if the free radicals are not kept under control, they are capable of damaging proteins, fats, and nucleic acids in the body. To help protect the cells and organ systems from the harmful effects of these reactive oxygen species, human beings need to support the detoxification functions of the body, which aid in limiting the amount of toxins (free radicals) that are present.

The liver is a primary organ of detoxification. **Phase I and Phase II** detoxification reactions take place primarily in the liver cells (hepatocytes). **Phase I detoxification** changes nonpolar chemicals that are not water-soluble into relatively polar, water-soluble compounds. Enzymes are required for this reaction and when grouped together, they are termed the cytochrome P-450 system. During Phase I detoxification reactions, there are toxic or reactive chemicals that form which are even more toxic than the original chemicals. **Phase II detoxification** is necessary therefore to add chemical groups to the toxic intermediates to

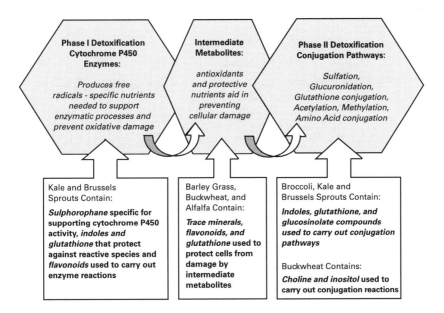

Figure 5.2

Vitamins, minerals, and phytonutrients found in kale, Brussels sprouts,
barley grass, buckwheat, and alfalfa that the liver uses to carry out phase I and
phase II detoxification, and to protect cells from oxidative damage by intermediate metabolites.

make them water-soluble. Once the toxic chemicals are water-soluble, they can be excreted via the kidneys. Phase I and Phase II detoxification pathways must remain functional for the proper removal of toxins from the body.

5.1.3 Removal or Excretion of Hormones

The endocrine glands secrete hormones that are excreted by the liver or are chemically altered to make them water-soluble so that the body may excrete them effectively. The steroid hormones that are altered by the liver include estrogen, cortisol, aldosterone, and thyroxin, among others. The liver detoxifies or excretes these hormones into the bile. If the liver is not functioning properly, there may be too many hormones in the body at one time, leading to overactivity. This excess of circulating hormones in the body will tax the endocrine system and cause other toxic reactions to occur.

5.1.4 Protein Metabolism

The ability of the liver to properly metabolize protein is critical to survival. The main functions of the liver in protein metabolism includes the manipulation and deamination of amino acids, the formation of plasma proteins, and the formation of urea so that ammonia can be removed from the body.

Ammonia is a toxic substance that is formed as a result of several metabolic processes in the body. The liver converts ammonia to urea, which is far less toxic than ammonia and is excreted in the urine. When there is decreased blood flow through the liver or the liver is malfunctioning in some way, the amount of ammonia in the blood stream increases and leads to hepatic coma and eventually death if the condition is not corrected.

5.1.5 Fat Metabolism

The liver played a central role in the synthesis of large amounts of cholesterol and phospholipids, the conversion of large amounts of proteins and carbohydrates into fats, the formation of most lipoproteins, and the metabolism of fatty acids (via oxidation).

The liver is also responsible for the metabolism and storage of carbohydrates, assimilation and storage of fat-soluble vitamins, and the storage of vitamins and minerals. Hence, it is essential that the liver remain in optimal working condition. However, toxins in the body can expose the liver to damage resulting in an inhibition of the cytochrome P450 system and/or a decrease in liver metabolism ("sluggish" liver). Symptoms of such toxic damage include fatigue, hormone imbalance, increased fat stores, headaches, and blurred vision, all associated with multiple health challenges.

Selected, scientifically validated, herbal medicines and foods (discussed in the latter part of this text) can aid in preventing damage to liver cells, and can promote the proper functioning of the liver detoxification pathways.

5.2 The Lungs

The lungs, above all other organs, have the greatest exposure to environmental conditions. Toxins in the form of gases, small solid particles, and liquid aerosols may enter the lungs and cause damage. The lungs can eliminate these toxic particles in three specific ways:

• **Impaction** allows large particles (>5 microns) to continue in straight paths through the airway passages landing primarily on the surfaces of the nose and throat or at the branching point of the airways. The process of impaction eliminates most toxic particles by encapsulating them in mucous, trapping them with cilia or hairs, and eliminating them via sneezing, swallowing, or blowing the nose. Failure of this mechanism can result in asthma or other respiratory ailments.

• **Sedimentation** allows medium-sized particles (1-5 microns) to deposit on a mucous layer in the peripheral airways of the lungs. These toxic particles are either exhaled or swallowed. If they are not removed in this way, they can reach the alveoli where they become trapped and cause permanent damage.

• **Diffusion** allows small toxic particles (< 0.1 microns) to enter into the lungs where they are either exhaled immediately or become trapped causing conditions such as lung disease (specifically asbestosis and silicosis).

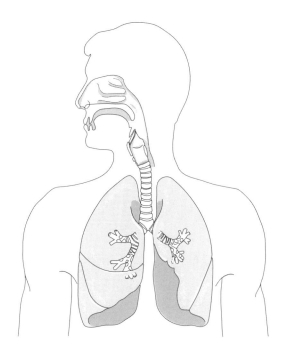

Figure 5.3
The Respiratory Tract

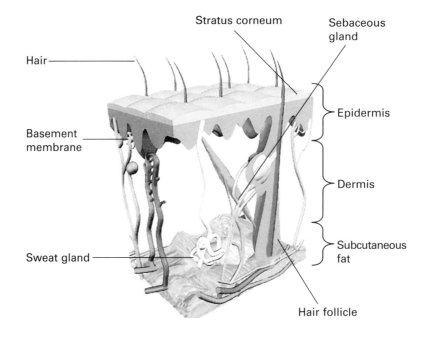

Figure 5.4
*The different layers of the skin maintain distinguishable
characteristics specific for supporting the purification process.*

While the lungs are equipped with their own barriers to protect the body from toxic overload, there are still multiple routes for toxic particles to enter the body. Thus, it is critical to maintain the health and functioning of all detoxification organs.

5.3 The Skin

The skin, or epidermis, is made up of an outer layer of epithelial cells and an inner layer referred to as the dermis. The epidermis contains several cell types. The **stratus corneum** constitutes the outermost protective boundary of the skin and is made up of dead skin cells. It is about one millimeter thick on average but varies in thickness in different parts of the body, thus offering some areas of the body more protection than others. Under the **stratus corneum** are living epidermal cells. **Melanocyte cells**, for example, produce melanin pigment that protects against ultraviolet injury, sunburn, and skin cancer. Melanin also quenches free radicals and gives skin its color. The other epidermal cells produce excretable lipids and keratin that protect the skin against water loss.

The **dermis layer** is composed largely of connective tissue. Collagen and elastin present in the dermis layer give skin its tensile strength and elasticity. The dermis also contains sebaceous glands located near hair follicles that secrete sebum. **Sebum** is a lipid mixture that has antibacterial and antifungal properties and helps to excrete lipid-soluble toxins from the body. Skin can detoxify in this way.

The rich blood supply of the dermis transports chemicals into the blood stream. Lipid soluble chemicals such as solvents, and caustic chemicals such as alkaline and acid solutions, can penetrate the stratus corneum, and if successful, will move through the epidermis and dermis. Multiple factors determine the amount of toxins absorbed through the skin. Oily solutions and organic solvents are easily absorbed due to the lipophilic properties of the stratus corneum. Injured skin, thin skin, wet skin, and thin plastic against skin (gloves) all allow chemicals to penetrate this barrier more readily and enter the blood stream.

Skin also contains cytochrome P450 enzymes that help to convert chemicals such as drugs, steroid hormones, and xenobiotics into more water-soluble forms that the body can more easily excrete.

5.4 The Intestinal Tract

The gastrointestinal tract functions as a critically important natural barrier, protecting the human body from harmful endogenous and exogenous toxins. The gastrointestinal system includes the entire alimentary tract (the mouth, parotid and salivary glands, esophagus, stomach, liver, gallbladder, pancreas, colon, small intestine and anus). The alimentary tract is responsible for several key functions in the body including:

- Absorption and regulation of water, electrolytes, and nutrients
- Protection from foreign microorganisms
- Digestion of food

The **small intestine** is responsible for digesting and absorbing nutrients, as well as serving as a barrier to toxic substances in the body. The **large intestine** houses a number of bacterial and dietary antigens (foreign substances) that are capable of forming systemic immune complexes if exposed to factors that should have been filtered out by the small intestine. It is crucial to protect the mucosal lining of the alimentary tract (particularly the large and small intestines) as any damage to it may result in the absorption of toxins, including bacteria and other pathogens.

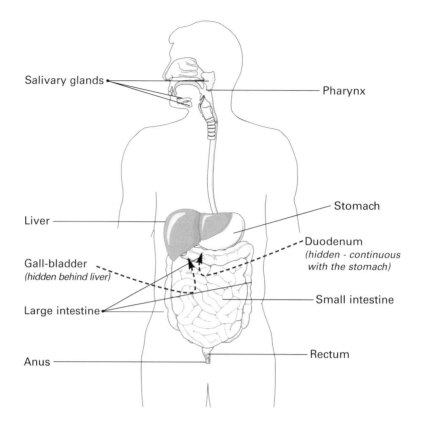

Figure 5.5
The Digestive Tract

There are specific endogenous and exogenous factors that contribute to the breakdown of the gastrointestinal system. Prolonged irritation to the lining of the gastrointestinal tract, nutritional insufficiencies, and exposure to bacterial endotoxins all may result in unfavorable changes in the permeability functions of the gastric mucosal lining. If the intestinal barrier does break down due to one of these causes, there is an increase in the number of larger molecules and antigenic substances that will permeate through the intestinal mucosa into the general circulation. This can contribute to the development of such conditions as irritable bowel syndrome, inflammatory bowel syndrome, food allergies, and autoimmune disorders such as rheumatoid arthritis. Other conditions that are common to an imbalance in gastrointestinal function include gas, diarrhea, diverticulitis, diverticulosis and constipation.

Substances that cause constipation include: analgesics, antacids, anti-diarrheal agents, antihistamines, anti-Parkinsonian drugs, diuretics, iron, chronic use of laxatives, opiates, tricyclic antidepressants, and some muscle relaxants. Constipation may predispose a person to hemorrhoids, diverticular disease, candidiasis, allergies, and colon cancer. Colon cancer is significantly related to chronic constipation, as the factors involved can be directly linked to a slow transit time (the amount of time it takes for food to pass through the intestinal tract).

There are key nutrients and herbs discussed in the following sections of this book that encourage the healthy functioning of the gastrointestinal tract, in order to prevent and treat constipation, and thereby reduce toxic exposure to this organ system.

Constipation is a condition associated with gastrointestinal dysfunction. It relates to the difficult or infrequent passage of stool, the hardness of stool, or a feeling of incomplete evacuation. If a person has less than three bowel movements per week, he/she is considered to be constipated.

Major causes of constipation include:

- Poor fluid intake
- Lack of exercise
- Mechanical obstruction
- Endocrine disorders
- Food allergies (commonly dairy)

- Low fiber diet
- Abnormal colon motility
- Neurological disorders
- Psychological disorders

Factors that influence the onset of colon cancer include[11,30] :

- Increased time of exposure to toxins in the colon
- Increased concentration of toxins along the colon wall
- Increased overall exposure to toxins in the colon

PART 1
CLINICAL REFERENCES

(CHAPTERS 1-5)

1. Angres, G. and M. Beth. 1991. Effects of dietary constituents on carcinogenesis in different tumor models: An overview from 1975 to 1988. *Cancer Nutr* 7: 337-486.
2. ATSDR. 1992. *Toxicological Profile for Cadmium*. U.S. Public Health Service, U.S. Department of Health and Human Services, Altanta, GA.
3. Belkin, M. and D. Fitzgerald. 1952. Tumor damaging capacity of plant materials. Plants used as cathartics. *J Natl Cancer Inst* 13: 139-155.
4. Blumenthal, M. et al. (Eds.). 2000. Herbal Medicine: Expanded Commission E Monographs. Austin, TX: American Botanical Council.
5. CAEPA. California EPA, Feb. 19, 1999. Office of Environmental Health Hazard Assessment. Chemicals on Candidate List for consideration under Proposition 65 due to high carcinogenicity concern.
6. Calabrese, E. J. and E. M. Kenyon. 1993. Air Toxics and Risk Assessment. Chelsea, MI: Lewis Publishers.
7. CAPCOA. 1994/1995. Air Toxics Hotspots Program Risk Assessment Guidance: Revised 1992 Risk Assessment Guidance and Draft Evaluation of Acute Non-Cancer Health Effects. California Environmental Protection Agency and California Air Pollution Control Officers Association. Berkeley, CA: Office of Environmental Health Hazard Assessment, CAEPA.
8. CDC October, 1991b. Centers for Disease Control. Preventing Lead Poisoning in Young Children. Atlanta, GA: U.S. Department of Health and Human Services, Public Health Service.
9. CDC. February, 1991a. Centers for Disease Control. Strategic Plan for the Elimination of Childhood Lead Poisoning. Atlanta, GA: U.S. Department of Health and Human Services, Public Health Service.
10. Chapin, R. E. and R. A. Sloane. 1997. NIEHS/NTP Reproductive Assessment by Continuous Breeding: Evolving Study Design and Summaries of Ninety Studies. *Environmental Health Perspectives* 105(1 Suppl): 199-394.
11. DiPalma, J. A. et al. 1991. Occupational and Industrial Toxin Exposures and the Gastrointestinal Tract. *Am J Gastroenterol* 86(9): 1107-1117. (Table 2: Selected Agents with Purported Digestive System Injury)
12. Dreosti, I. E. 1998. Nutrition, cancer, and aging. *Ann NY Acad Sci* 854: 371-377.
13. EPA. 1993. Integrated Risk Information System (IRIS) on Cadmium. Environmental Criteria and Assessment Office, Office of Health and Environmental Assessment. Cincinnati, OH: Office of Research and Development.
14. EPA. 1997. Health Effects Assessment Summary Tables. FY 1997 Update. Office of Research and Development, Office of Emergency and Remedial Response,Washington, DC. EPA-540-R-97-036.
15. EPA. 1999. List of Chemicals Evaluated for Carcinogenic Potential (8/25/99). Washington, DC: Office of Pesticide Programs.
16. Eriksson, M. et al. 1990. Exposure to dioxins as a risk factor for soft tissue sarcoma: A population-based case-control study. *J Natl Cancer Inst* 82: 486-490.
17. Ernst, M. et al. 1998. Immune cell functions in industrial workers after exposure to 2,3,7,8-tetrachlorodibenzo-p dioxin: Dissociation of antigen-specific T-cell responses in cultures of diluted whole blood and of isolated peripheral blood mononuclear cells. Environ Health Perspect 106(2 Suppl): 701-705.
18. Eskenazi, B. et al. 1998. Seveso women's health study: A study of the effects of TCDD on reproductive health. *Organohalogen compounds* 38: 219-222.
19. Esteller, M. et al. 1997. Germ line polymorphisms in cytochrome P450IA1 (C4887 CYP IA1) and methylenetetrahydrofolate reductase (MTHFR) genes and endometrial cancer susceptibility. *Carcinogenesis* 18: 2307-2311.
20. Fernandez-Salguero, P. M. and F. J. Gonzalez. 1996. Targeted disruption of specific cytochromes P450 and xenobiotic receptor genes. *Methods Enzymol* 272: 412-430.
21. Fingerhut, M. A. et al. 1991 Cancer mortality in workers exposed to 2,3,7,8 tetrachlorodibenzo-p-dioxin. *N Engl J Med* 324(4): 212-218.
22. Flesch-Janys, D. et al. 1999. Epidemiological investigation of breast cancer incidence in a cohort of female workers with high exposure to PCDD/CDF and HCH. *Organohalogen Compounds* 44:379-382.
23. Flodstrom, S. and U. G. Ahlborg. 1992. Relative tumor promoting activity of some polychlorinated dibenzo-p-dioxin-, dibenzofuran-, and biphenyl congeners in female rats. *Chemosphere* 25:1(2):169-172.
24. Foldeak, S. and G. Dombradi. 1964. Tumor-growth inhibiting substances of plant origin. Isolation of the active principle of Arctium lappa. *Acta Phys Chem* 10: 91-93.
25. Gasiewicz, T. A. 1997. Dioxins and the AhR: probes to uncover processes in neuroendocrine development. *Neurotoxicology* 18: 393-414.

26. Hardy, M. P. et al. 2000. A metabolite of methoxychlor, 2,2-bis(p-hydroxyphenyl)-1,1,1-trichloroethane, reduces testosterone biosynthesis in rat leydig cells through suppression of steady-state messenger ribonucleic acid levels of the cholesterol side-chain cleavage enzyme. *Biol Reprod* 62(3): 571-578.

27. Kimbrough, R. D. et al. 1977. Epidemiology and pathology of a tetrachlorodlibenzodioxin poisoning episode. *Arch Environ Health* 32(2): 77-86.

28. Klaassen, C. et al. (eds.). 1996. Casarett and Doull's Toxicology. The Basic Science of Poisons, 5th Ed. New York: Pergamon Press. (Table 13-2: Types of Hepatic Injury).

29. Kouri, R. E. et al. 1974. Aryl hydrocarbon hydroxylase inductlon in human lymphocyte cultures by 2,3,7,8-tetrachlorodibenzo-p-dioxin. Life Sci 15(9): 1585-1595.

30. Malachowsky, M. J. 1995. Health Effects of Toxic Substances. Rockville, MD: Government Institutes.

31. Manson, J. 1996. Teratogens. In Klaassen, C. et al. (eds.). 1996. Casarett and Doull's Toxicology. The Basic Science of Poisons, 5th Ed. New York: Pergamon Press. Chapter

32. Massanyi, P. et al. 1998. Reproductive Toxicity of Cadmium. Presented at INABIS '98 - 5th Internet World Congress on Biomedical Sciences at McMaster University, Canada, Dec 7-16th, 1998.

33. Mills, S. 1994. The Complete Guide to Modern Herbalism. Great Britain: Thorsons.

34. Morita, K. et al. 1984. A desmutagenic factor isolated from burdock (Arctium lappa Linne). *Mutat Res* 129(1): 25-31.

35. OEHHA. October, 1997. Draft Technical Support Document for the Determination of Noncancer Chronic Reference Exposure Levels. Office of Environmental Health Hazard Assessment, California Environmental Protection Agency.

36. Prenney, B. April, 1987. The Massachusetts Lead Program: Moving Toward Phase 2. Prevention Update. Developed by the Maternal and Child Health Consortium Project and the National Coalition on Prevention of Mental Retardation.

37. Rabinowitz, M. and H. Needleman. 1983. Petrol Lead Sales and Umbilical Cord Blood Lead Levels in Boston, MA. *Lancet* 8314/5 (1): 63.

38. Roth, G. S. et al. 2000. Effects of reduced energy intake on the biology of aging: The primate model. *Eur J Clin Nutr* 54 Suppl 3: S15-S20.

39. Schardein, J. 1985. Chemically Induced Birth Defects. New York: Dekker.

40. Sigerist H. E. 1951. A History of Medicine, vols. I and II. New York: Oxford University Press.

41. Tarcher, A.1992. Principles and practice of environmental medicine. New York: Plenum Medical Book Co.

42. USDHHS. 1993. U.S. Department of Health and Human Services. Registry of Toxic Effects of Chemical Substances. National Toxicology Information Program. Bethesda, MD: National Library of Medicine.

43. USDHHS. July, 1998. U.S. Department of Health and Human Services, Public Health Service, Agency for Toxic Substances and Disease Registry. The Nature and Extent of Lead Poisoning in the United States: A Report to Congress.

44. Vander, A. et al. 1985. Human Physiology. New York: McGraw-Hill Book Co.

45. Walters, R. 1993. Options: The Alternative Cancer Therapy Book. Garden City Park, NY: Avery Publishing Group.

46. Weindruch, R. et al. 1986. The retardation of aging in mice by dietary restriction: longevity, cancer, immunity and lifetime energy intake. *J Nutr* 116(4): 641-654.

47. Weindruch, R. 1992. Effect of caloric restriction on age-associated cancers. *Exp Gerontol* 27(5-6): 575-581.

PART 2

NUTRITIONAL AND BOTANICAL
OPTIONS FOR CLINICAL PURIFICATION

SCIENTIFIC MONOGRAPHS

"Vitamins are better assimilated if taken [as] food.
No synthetic principle is as good as the real thing..."
–Cayce

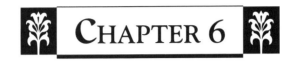

CHAPTER 6

CALORIC RESTRICTION

6

CALORIC RESTRICTION

6.1 Description

Caloric restriction without malnutrition is the only proven method to date that slows the human aging process and extends life span, while also improving health and well being.[348] Researchers have been stating this once theoretical notion as fact for well over 60 years.[26,159,368]

6.2 Possible Mechanisms of Action

• Dietary restriction reduces the number of reactive oxidant molecules in the body.[116,380] While numerous mechanisms have been proposed for the observed long-term health benefits of caloric restriction,[117,369,380,381] the free radical theory is the most widely accepted. Dietary restriction modulates many key aspects of free radical metabolism, including free radical generation, lipid peroxidation, DNA damage, and the cytosolic cellular defense systems.[380] This theory offers a solid explanation for the following observed biochemical and physiologic phenomena[382] :

• The inverse relationship between basal metabolic rate and average lifespan in mammals
• The connection between increased incidences of degenerative diseases in the latter part of life and the accumulation of oxidative damage over time
• The demonstrated health benefits of dietary restriction
• Greater longevity of females
• The increase in autoimmune dysfunctions with age

6.3 Caloric Restriction and Mitochondria

Cellular mitochondria are vulnerable to oxidative damage that occurs because of diet, disease, and the aging process. Partly, this vulnerability stems from the fact that most oxidative metabolic reactions take place in the mitochondria. Mitochondria are considered to be the "power houses" of cells, producing energy in the form of adenosine triphosphate (ATP), but they are also the storage sheds for reactive oxygen species (ROS). ROS are most concentrated in the membranes of the mitochondria where they have direct access to DNA, the key generator of this critical metabolic machinery. Damage to mitochondria by oxidants creates an inefficient metabolic mechanism that worsens over time, ultimately increasing free radical output. This free radical output causes damage to proteins, lipids, and DNA throughout the cell and as cells become less efficient, so do the organs and tissues they comprise. The organs and tissues, in turn, become less able to cope with free radical attacks, which leads to aging. **Caloric restriction lowers free radical production in the mitochondria and many scientists believe that this is the mechanism by which caloric restriction slows the aging process.**[369]

Research scientists are stating with conviction that a diet containing adequate essential nutrients and a caloric input that minimizes random free radical reactions in the body will increase a healthy human lifespan by five to ten years.[116]

According to Yu[380] :   **Dietary restriction is widely recognized to be the most effective means of intervening in the aging process...**

5 Year Values for:	Normal Diet: 688 calories per day	Reduced Diet: 477 calories per day
Body weight	31 pounds	21 pounds
Percent of weight from fat	25%	10%
Measures of Health		
Blood pressure (systole/diastole)	129/60	121/51
Serum glucose level (mg/dL)	71	56
Serum insulin level (μU/mL)	93	29
Serum triglycerides (mg/dL)	169	67

Table 6.1
Results of an ongoing trial of caloric restriction in rhesus monkeys.[369] *Table represents data at five years.*

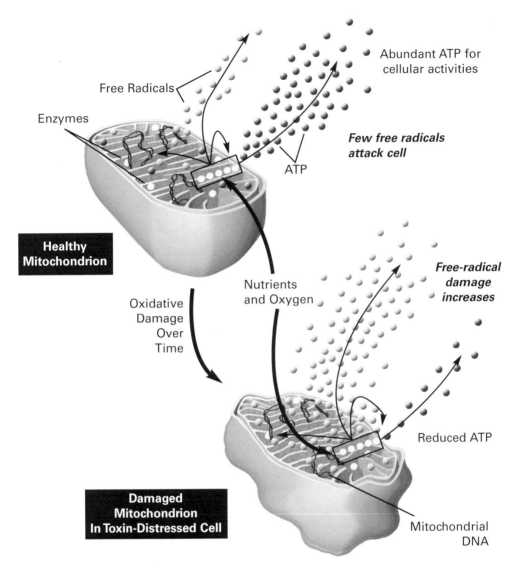

Figure 6.1

Healthy mitochondrion versus unhealthy mitochondrion damaged by free radicals.

The notable positive benefits of dietary restriction mandate a nutritious diet, not simply a reduction in caloric intake. Because a nutritious restricted diet may be difficult to follow in our fast-paced society, dietary supplements can play a role by providing essential nutrient complexes that might be lacking in a reduced-calorie diet. In addition, many of these complexes have tertiary functions, providing additional health benefits, as described later in this book.

6.4 Research

6.4.1 Dietary Restriction and Cancer

A long-term study by Frankel et al[94] examined the correlation between childhood energy intake (recorded in the 1937-1939 Lord Boyd Orr's Carnegie Survey of Family Diet and Health) and adult mortality from cancer. After controlling for smoking and other non-dietary causes of cancer, this study demonstrated a direct correlation between high-energy intake in childhood and the development of cancer later in life. Clearly, a healthy, calorie-restricted diet in childhood can reduce cancer risk in adulthood.

Clinically, dietary restriction in humans was shown to suppress urinary biomarkers of oxidative DNA base damage, reflecting a decrease in the level of DNA damage in cells (Table 6.2).[300]

Date (1989/90):	May 5	July 18	July 27	Aug19	Aug 30	Jan 8	Jan 18
Caloric intake (kcal/day)	2,000	2,100	1,200	2,000	1,200	2,200	1,100
Body weight (lbs)	180	180	175	180	173	181	173
Thymidine glycol (dRTg) (nmoles/kg/day)	0.26	0.27	0.11	0.19	0.10	0.28	0.11
8-hydroxydeoxyguanosine (8-dRG-OH) (nmoles/kg/day)	0.35	0.40	0.08	0.30	0.16	0.33	0.09

Table 6.2
Urinary biomarkers of oxidative DNA base damage (UBODBD) for a male subject in his 50's as a function of low and high dietary caloric intake.[300] Measurements were taken after 10 days of constant daily caloric intake.

In another study, caloric restriction in obese human subjects resulted in reduced rectal cell proliferation, an intermediate biomarker in colon carcinogenesis.[313]

In a study of experimental mammary cancer in rats, caloric restriction correlated linearly with prolongation of latency to palpable carcinomas and a reduction in final incidence of mammary cancer.[393] This experimental case may validate the potential use of caloric restriction to inhibit the conversion of precancerous cells to malignant cells. In this study, caloric restriction also correlated with an increase in cortical steroid levels that explained 95% of the linear relationship between cancer and dietary restriction. Thus, dietary restriction may offer some chemoprotection by normalizing adrenal function.

6.4.2 Dietary Restriction and Free Radicals

In diet-restricted rats, free radical damage as measured by thiobarbituric acid-reactive material and lipofuscin accumulation was much lower than in rats fed *ad libitum*.[265] In liver tissue, the expression of superoxide dismutase and catalase typically decreases with age in *ad libitum* fed rats. However, in diet-restricted rats these antioxidant enzymes were significantly elevated even at 21 and 28 months of age. Glutathione peroxidase was also elevated at 28 months of age. This result has been supported by additional research[174,257] in which glutathione reductase, glutathione S-transferase, and catalase enzyme activities were essentially unchanged in diet restricted rats at 24 months while the levels in *ad libitum* fed rats steadily declined from 12 to 24 months of age. These studies suggest that the beneficial effects of dietary restriction result from the preservation of antioxidant enzyme activity in animals.

Some researchers argue that dietary restriction inhibits the generation of oxidative molecules and does not directly increase antioxidant enzyme activity. Gong et al[107] reported an apparent reduction in antioxidant enzyme activity in rat lens and kidney in response to dietary restriction, presumably due to a decrease in substrate oxidative molecules. Dietary restriction at various ages in the rat decreases the formation of superoxide and hydroxyl radicals, and hydrogen peroxide in liver microsomes.[180] Additionally, mitochondrial resting respiratory rates in brain, heart, and kidney tissues remain constant with age in diet restricted rats while they progressively rise in controls, with a corresponding rise in superoxide radical and hydrogen peroxide generation in the latter.[305] The latter result supports the mitochondrial hypothesis in that dietary restriction successfully maintained the resting respiratory rate, showing that this method keeps the mitochondria functioning efficiently over time.

Unmistakably, dietary restriction offers substantial health benefits due to its effect on modulating the production and metabolism of reactive oxygen species, or free radicals. Supplementation with whole food complexes that are naturally rich in antioxidants in the restricted diet may provide additional health benefits. Epidemiological and clinical studies have revealed roles for antioxidants in the age-associated decline of immune function and the reduction of risk from cancer and heart disease.[213] In combination, dietary restriction and supplementation of the diet with select nutrient complexes can both slow the aging process and reduce the incidence of "secondary" age-associated pathologies.

6.4.3 Dietary Restriction and Gastroprotection

Dietary restriction renders rats more resistant to experimental gastric mucosal injury induced by aspirin or acidified ethanol.[181] The restricted diet prevents the relative decrease in mucosal glutathione and energy stores (ATP) that normally occurs with gastric mucosal injuries in the aging population.

6.4.4 Dietary Restriction and Cardioprotection

In a study in which rats were subjected to a calorie restricted diet and/or endurance exercise for 18.5 months, cardiac mitochondria showed decreased malondialdehyde levels indicative of a decrease in lipid peroxidative damage under all experimental conditions relative to controls.[162] Dietary restriction also increased the antioxidant enzymes superoxide dismutase, Se-dependent glutathione peroxidase, and glutathione S-transferase in cardiac cytosol.

6.4.5 Dietary Restriction and Kidney Function

The ratio of reduced glutathione to oxidized glutathione signifies the level of oxidative stress occurring in an organ. Caloric and carbohydrate restriction in mice during eight weeks of their growing phase significantly increased the ratio of reduced glutathione to oxidized glutathione, indicating a reduction in oxidative stress in the kidney.[44] When carbohydrate was substituted with non-nutritive bulk in the diet, glutathione peroxidase and cytochrome oxidase

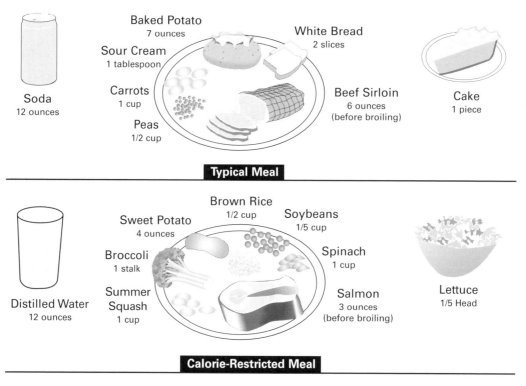

Figure 6.2
Graphic representation of a typical meal in comparison to a caloric restricted meal.

activities increased significantly and the *in vivo* peroxidation by the kidney tissue markedly decreased. These results illustrate how caloric restriction can increase enzymatic decomposition of hydroperoxide free radicals and decrease oxidative stress in the kidney.

6.4.6 Dietary Restriction and Humans

A clinical study on the effects of dietary restriction was performed on four men and four women housed in Biosphere 2, a closed ecological space of 7 million cubic feet near Tucson, Arizona. As a result of poor food yields, the inhabitants of the biosphere consumed a low-calorie but nutrient dense diet for their two-year stay in the habitat. The men and women showed 18% and 10% weight loss, respectively. Further, the researchers measured blood lipids, glucose, insulin, glycosylated hemoglobin and renin during and following the experiment. The human subjects' blood profiles improved significantly in all parameters that were measured, clearly demonstrating that humans react similarly to other vertebrates when subject to a calorie restricted diet.[357]

6.5 Overview

These clinical results coupled with the results of earlier trials strongly suggest that **dietary restriction**:

- Reduces free radical-induced mitochondrial damage
- Increases levels of antioxidant enzymes and free-radical scavengers
- Reduces DNA damage and the risk of cancer
- Inhibits carcinogenesis
- Improves kidney function by reducing oxidative stress on the organ
- Improves cardiac function and inhibits lipid peroxidation in cardiac mitochondria
- Protects the gastrointestinal tract from mucosal injury
- Has similar effects in humans as with other mammals

6.5.1 Administration of Dietary Restriction

Most animal studies use a regime of 30-40% caloric restriction, however as little at 10-20% can have positive benefits.[369] Figure 1.2 illustrates a potential calorie-restricted meal of nutrient dense foods with respect to a typical meal.

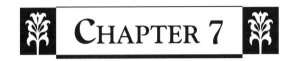

CHAPTER 7

CAYENNE PEPPER

Capsicum spp.

7

Cayenne Pepper

Capsicum spp.

7.1 Description and Medical History

Cayenne pepper (*Capsicum*) is native to tropical America and has been used by Native Americans as a medicinal food for at least nine thousand years.[61] Based on archeological evidence, its cultivation in Mexico began around seven thousand years ago. Christopher Columbus brought the pepper plant to Europe from the New World.[30,183,249] Today this fruit is cultivated throughout the world for its nutritional and pharmacological properties.[186,370] *Capsicum annuum* is an annual or biennial plant,[138] while *C. frutescens* is a perennial shrub. The fruits and seeds are the commonly used elements.

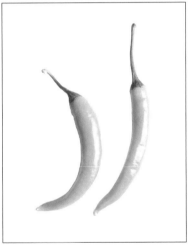

Figure 7.1
Capsicum spp. (Cayenne pepper)

7.2 Known Medicinal Constituents

Cayenne pepper's pungent nature has captured the attention of physicians, researchers, and connoisseurs throughout history.[28,30,42,70,153,212,230,249,296,365] The compounds responsible for its pungent nature, namely, capsaicin, dihydrocapsaicin, and their derivatives, possess well-documented health benefits. The fruit's degree of pungency, calculated in Scoville (heat) units, determines its primary use as a potent medicine, a functional food, or an accessory spice. In 1912, William Scoville, a Detroit pharmacologist, measured capsaicin by having a panel of hardy souls sip a sweetened solution of dried chile peppers dissolved in alcohol.

The concoction had decreasing amounts of capsaicin until it no longer burned. The results were successfully converted into Scoville units, though no one is quite sure what happened to the tasters. A chemical process has replaced this subjective test, although the results are still expressed as Scoville units. Scoville units can range from zero to more than half a million.[374]

The following list includes cayenne pepper's tertiary functional components, including those responsible for its pungency, in addition to its primary nutritional components:

- Capsaicinoids (0.05-1.5%): *phenolic amides, largely capsaicin, dihydrocapsaicin, and their derivatives*
- Steroidal alkaloids, including solanidine and flavonoids
- Carotenoids: *carotene and capsanthin*
- Vitamins A and C, proteins, and coumarins
- Trace volatile oils

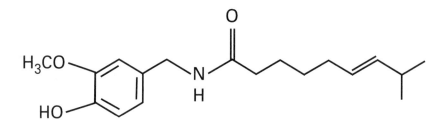

Figure 7.2
Molecular structure of trans-capsaicin.

7.3 Indications for Use

Healthcare practitioners use the fruit, both internally and externally, to treat numerous conditions including arthritis, bleeding, chills, colds, coughs, digestive disorders, dysentery, headache, high cholesterol, migraine headaches, pain, poor circulation, and sinus congestion.[30,58,186,320,354]   The pepper's primary indications for use, that are substantiated by research, include:

- Clinical purification[154,173,210,230,296,344,345]
- Peripheral circulatory insufficiency[173,210,344,345]
- Gastric disorders, including poor appetite and digestion, atonic dyspepsia, gastric flatulence, impaired gastric secretion, and peptic ulcer.[1,151,152,188,330]

Caution: There is a small amount of evidence that suggests large amounts of capsaicin may impair healing of acute gastric mucosal damage.[252]

- Migraines and cluster headaches[202,299]
- Elevated plasma triglycerides and free fatty acids[278,308]
- Depressed immune function[383]
- Superfluous fat and obesity [72,158,187,211,220,379]
- Zosteriform herpes simplex II (shingles) and genital herpes -to inhibit the spread of the infection.[33,310]
- Myalgias and Neuralgias[195,252]

7.4 Mechanisms of Action

- Cayenne is a thermogenic agent as it stimulates metabolism and aids in weight loss.[72,158,187,211,220,379]   It also stimulates adrenal catecholamine secretion (primarily epinephrine)[15,158,362] and vasodilation, consequently promoting peripheral circulation.[173,210,344,345]

Specifically, cayenne has the following internal and external mechanisms of action:

Internal

- Capsaicin stimulates perfusion of gastric mucosa, facilitating digestion and gastric healing.[152,188,377]   Cayenne also has been shown to improve intestinal transit time in humans.[131,48] Dietary capsaicin and several other spices prominently enhanced pancreatic lipase activity in rats.[260]

- Topically, capsaicin stimulates the internal release of substance P and calcitonin gene-related peptide (CGRP) in sensory afferent fibers innervating vascular and glandular smooth muscle. These neurotransmitters appear to mediate the initial vasodilatory effect.[173,210,344,345] Sicuteri et al[299] discovered that capsicum alleviates the symptoms associated with migraines and cluster headaches and proposed that this therapeutic action is due to capsicum's vasodilatory effects.

- Capsaicin incites catecholamine (epinephrine) production from the adrenal medulla, stimulating metabolism.[15,158,362]

External

- Applied to skin, capsaicin depletes substance P (involved in pain transduction) from unmyelinated C-afferent sensory nerves, giving rise to its analgesic (desensitization) effects in myalgias and neuralgias.[195,240]

7.5 Research

7.5.1 Capsicum and Chemoprotection

Surh et al[317] conducted a review of the literature on capsicum's inhibitory activity in cancer initiation and promotion. The literature supports an anticancer role for capsaicinoids, the active components of red pepper, as anti-inflammatory and antioxidant compounds inhibiting cell membrane oxidative pathways that lead to carcinogen and mutagen activation. Table 7.1 summarizes the findings of research prior to 1998.

The bulk of research on capsaicin's chemoprotective effects has focused on inhibition of xenobiotic metabolizing enzymes. Capsaicin has a direct inhibitory effect on the cytochrome P450-dependent monooxygenase biochemical pathways involved in enzymatic detoxification. Overstimulation of Phase I enzymes can lead to accumulation of harmful intermediates. Capsaicin suppresses the activity of rat epidermal aryl hydrocarbon hydroxylase linked to the cytochrome P450 1A isoform responsible for the metabolism and subsequent mutagenicity of benzo[a]pyrene[218] Capsaicin also appears to stimulate apoptosis in numerous transformed cell lines *in vitro* and *in vivo* via inhibition of plasma membrane NADH oxidase[224,225] supporting an antioxidative role for the chemical. NADH oxidase also mediates the oxidative burst response of macrophages to antigens that results in release of toxic oxygen species. Capsaicin inhibits the oxidative burst via a calcium-dependent mechanism involving calmodulin.[279,285] In addition, Bcl-2 and the protein phosphatase, calcineurin, appear to be involved in capsaicin-induced apoptosis[373] Red pepper extract was shown to be an inducer of the anti-carcinogenic enzyme quinone reductase in mouse liver cells *in vitro*[324] and chili extracts decreased the mutagenicity of urban air samples *in vitro*.[83]

These findings strongly suggest that capsaicin can inhibit the initiating activities of certain chemical carcinogens via modulation of their metabolism.[317] Capsaicin also shows chemoprotective activity in the post-initiation stage.[139,224,225,317] Capsaicin repressed the growth

Summary of Results	Test Model
Capsaicin inhibition of cytochrome P450 1A2 (CYP 1A2) correlated with antimutagenic activity against selected heterocyclic amines.[329]	Hamster liver microsomes; *in vitro*; Capsaicin administered orally
Oral administration of capsaicin to Syrian gold hamsters inhibited NNK metabolism, specifically a-hydroxylation, in hepatic and pulmonary microsomes.[392]	Hamster hepatic and pulmonary microsomes
Intraperitoneal administration of capsaicin attenuated cyclophosphamide-induced chromosomal aberrations and DNA breaks in mice.[68]	Mouse; *in vivo*
Capsaicin and dihydrocapsaicin inhibited the mutagenicity and tumorigenicity of vinyl carbamate and dimethyl nitrosamine, which are preferentially activated by CYP 2E1.[316]	*Salmonella typhimurium*; *in vitro*; Mouse; *in vivo* (topical)
Chili extracts inhibited mutagenic activity of urban air samples in nitroreductase and O-acetyltransferase active bacteria.[83]	*Salmonella typhimurium*; *in vitro*; Chili extract
Capsaicin inhibited hamster microsome-mediated mutagenicity of tobacco-specific nitrosamine (NNK) in bacteria.[328]	Hamster microsome-mediated mutagenicity; *Salmonella typhimurium*; *in vitro*
Capsaicin inhibited NADPH-dependent carbonyl reduction and α-hydroxylation of NNK by hamster hepatic microsomes. Inhibition determined by analysis of testosterone metabolites for CYP 3A1, 2A2, 2B1, 2B2, 2C6, and 2C11.[391]	Hamster hepatic microsomes; *in vitro*
Capsaicin ameliorated peroxidative damage to rat liver and lung due to chloroform, carbon tetrachloride and dichloromethane via inhibition of CYP 2E1 peroxidative metabolism.[67]	Rat; *in vivo*
Capsaicin inhibited S9 mediated metabolism and subsequent covalent DNA binding of aflatoxin B1.[327]	Rat liver enzyme S9; *in vitro*
Capsaicin pretreatment protected against free radical-induced pulmonary damage in rats exposed to gaseous chemical irritants (SO2 and NO2).[66]	Rat; *in vivo*
Capsaicin inhibited activity of rat epidermal aryl hydrocarbon hydroxylase linked to the cytochrome P450 1A isoform, thus inhibiting subsequent metabolism and covalent DNA binding of mutagen benzo[a]pyrene.[218]	Mouse and human keratinocytes; *in vitro*
Note: CYP=cytochrome P450	

Table 7.1

Summary of research on chemoprotective effects of capsicum/capsaicin.[317]

of a number of human and animal cancer cell lines[224,225] and direct injection of capsaicin significantly reduced melanoma tumor growth in mice.[225]

7.5.2 Capsicum and Lipid Metabolism

In vitro studies on the antioxidant activity of capsaicin suggest it inhibits lipid peroxidation. Thus, it may protect against the deleterious cross-linking of proteins, DNA damage, and production of inflammatory molecules induced by lipid peroxidation. Capsaicin, was shown to inhibit lipid peroxidation in rat liver microsomes with a dose-dependency and effect comparable with the strong chemical antioxidants BHA and BHT.[262]

The mechanism responsible for capsaicin's lipid antioxidant activity is not well understood. It may act by scavenging the reactive oxygen species that initiate lipid peroxidation[115,263] or, as many researchers hypothesize, it may chelate metal ions needed for initiation of lipid peroxidation, as has been shown for other spice principles.[136,231,262] The alkyl side chain of capsaicin may be involved in the regeneration of antioxidants during peroxidation, as is the case with vitamin E.[145] Additionally, capsaicin accumulates in the liver where it binds covalently and irreversibly to hepatic macromolecular proteins potentially involved in lipid oxidative pathways.[215]

In vivo, red pepper fed to rats on a high cholesterol diet significantly lowered liver cholesterol accumulation and increased the fecal excretion of free cholesterol and bile acids[281] (Table 7.2). In this study, dietary red pepper, but not purified capsaicin, also lowered serum cholesterol levels suggesting the presence of other hypocholesterolemic factors in whole red pepper. In another study, rats fed capsaicin or capsicum extract for 60 days showed marked reductions in body weight, blood urea nitrogen, blood glucose, phospholipids, triglycerides, total cholesterol, free fatty acids, glutamic pyruvic transaminase, and alkaline phosphatase, as well as some hyperemia of liver tissue[220] (Table 7.3). Cholesterol crystal nucleation in a model bile was inhibited by low molecular weight biliary proteins from rats fed capsaicin as compared with controls.[135]

7.5.3 Gastrointestinal Effects of Capsicum

The ingestion of chili pepper is associated with a faster whole gut transit time in humans.[164] However, it has been shown that while gastric emptying was faster in humans after ingestion of 400 mg of capsaicin,[69] the orocecal (intestinal) transit was slower in humans after ingestion of 2 grams of red pepper[348] (Table 7.4). The experimental protocols in these studies were markedly different. Thus, the net effect of red pepper on the rate of gastrointestinal transit is still unclear.

Results

	Basal control diet	1% Cholesterol diet	1% Cholesterol diet + 5 mg red pepper	1% Cholesterol diet + 15 mg natural capsaicin	1% Cholesterol diet + 15 mg synthetic capsaicin
Liver Cholesterol					
Total	4.48±0.27	11.37±0.37	8.34±0.23 (P<0.001)	8.91±0.65 (P<0.01)	9.25±0.23 (P<0.001)
Free	1.81±0.03	4.9±0.18	4.95±0.17	5.46±0.16	4.69±0.31
Ester	2.67±0.25	6.42±0.48	3.39±0.29 (P<0.001)	3.45±0.52 (P<0.001)	4.56±0.31 (P<0.01)
Serum Cholesterol					
Total	113.0±6.93	176.0±8.32	138.0±6.07 (P<0.01)	196.0±7.39	181.0±8.88
Free	28.0±1.84	60.0±5.63	53.0±2.08	73.0±8.31	61.0±7.25
Ester	85.0±5.89	116.0±4.76	85.0±7.58 (P<0.01)	123.0±9.44	120.0±9.59
Free Cholesterol and Bile Acids in Fecal Excretions					
Free Chol.	4.79±0.34	18.33±1.71	27.33±1.65 (P<0.01)	25.33±0.82 (P<0.01)	25.05±0.84 (P<0.01)
Cholic Acid	1.03±0.05	1.69±0.11	2.3±0.13 (P<0.01)	1.96±0.13	1.89±0.15
Deoxy-cholic acid	0.88±0.06	1.63±0.09	2.64±0.14 (P<0.001)	2.06±0.15 (P<0.05)	2.13±0.17 (P<0.05)
Total bile acids	1.91±0.11	3.32±0.18	4.94±0.26 (P<0.001)	4.02±0.27 (P<0.05)	4.02±0.30 (P<0.05)

Table 7.2

Effect of red pepper/capsaicin on liver and serum cholesterol levels and fecal excretion of free cholesterol and bile acids in rats fed exogenous cholesterol diets for seven weeks.[281]

Results

	Total Cholesterol (mg/100mL)	Triglycerides	Free Fatty Acids	Phospholipids
Saline	125.0±13.4	162.0±17.4	590.0±50.2	180.0±19.2
Capsaicin (50 mg/kg BW/day)	87.6±3.5 (P<0.005)	141.3±12.1 (P<0.05)	504.6±11.5 (P<0.005)	144.1±8.9 (P<0.005)

Note: Data shown are for measurements taken on day 60. All rats had free access to food and water throughout the experimental period.

Table 7.3

Plasma chemical results in rats fed capsaicin via stomach tube for 60 days vs. saline fed controls.[220]

In anesthetized rats, varying doses of capsaicin delivered to the gastric lumen increased blood flow (hyperemia) and acid secretion of the gastric mucosa.[188] An *in vitro* study using a human ileocecal carcinoma cell line suggests that red pepper extract increases the permeability of intestinal epithelial cells for ions and macromolecules.[142] **These studies suggest that red pepper may enhance gastrointestinal function, aiding in digestion and the elimination of toxins.**

Results	
OCTT (min) **Before Red Pepper**	**OCTT (min)** **After Red Pepper (2g, powder)**
88 (n=16)	128 (n=16)(P<0.01)

Table 7.4
The effect of red pepper ingestion on Orocecal Transit Time (OCTT).[348]

There is substantial evidence that red pepper protects the intestine from chemically and physically induced damage in humans (Table 7.5) and animals[150,152,330,377] and chili use is inversely correlated with the incidence of peptic ulcer in humans.[151]

The effect of red pepper on gastric function likely involves capsaicin-sensitive sensory nerves that may secrete peptides that enhance the microcirculation in the gastric mucosa.[1,252] These neurons may contribute to repair processes and limit the inflammatory response to injury.

Results	
Study Group	**Aggregate** **Endoscopic Lesion Score (0-4)**
Control (n=18)	4
Chili (n=18)	1.5 (P<0.05)

Table 7.5
The chemoprotective effect of dietary chili pepper ingestion against aspirin-induced gastroduodenal damage in human subjects as measured by endoscopic lesion score.[377]

7.5.4 Antimicrobial Action of Capsaicin.

Cichewicz et al[58] performed a survey of the Mayan herbal pharmacopoeia and found a number of herbal remedies directed at ailments of probable microbial origin. Most of the remedies list capsicum fruit, alone or in conjunction with the leaves, roots, or seeds, as the main ingredient and these were applied to a variety of ailments, including respiratory problems, bowel complaints, earaches, and sores. Many of the remedies called for boiling or heating of the medicinal mixture before administration suggesting that the putative antimicrobial activity is resistant to heat. In addition, Huastec Mayans have reported using fresh and heated capsicum to treat infected wounds and fresh burns.[12]

The researchers examined the potential antimicrobial activity of 11 varieties of capsicum species on 16 bacteria and yeast strains. Untreated and boiled (20 minutes) extracts were tested and the researchers examined the microbial strains for inhibition or stimulation of growth *in vitro* using a common filter disk assay. The researchers did not examine the cytotoxicity of the extracts on the microbial strains. Purified capsaicinoids (capsaicin and dihydrocapsaicin) from a commercial source showed no growth inhibition, suggesting that these constituents are not responsible for the reported antimicrobial action of capsicum.

Table 7.6 summarizes the results of this experiment for the fruit extracts of *Capsicum annuum* varieties. The researchers also tested leaf extracts in some cases. However, the leaves of Solanaceous plants (nightshade family of which capsicum is a member) are known to be toxic and should not be used medicinally without consulting a physician.

The capsicum extracts were shown to be growth-inhibitory on three of the 16 microbial species tested. *Clostridium spp.* are common anaerobic bacteria often found in soil, sewage, aquatic sediments, and decaying organic matter, as well as in the intestines of animals.[13] *C. tetani* is the bacterium responsible for tetanus and *C. botulinum* (not tested) causes botulism. *Streptococcus pyogenes* is the central pathogen identified in a variety of cutaneous and systemic infections. Thus, capsicum extracts do appear to have some valuable antimicrobial activity. Although, the activity is not global as capsicum actually stimulated growth in some species, such as the *Bacillus* strains tested. However, a later study has shown that capsaicin strongly inhibits growth of *B. subtilis*.[219]

7.6 Overview

These clinical results coupled with the results of earlier trials strongly suggest that **cayenne pepper:**

- Inhibits oxidative pathways involved in cancer initiation and promotion
- Reduces liver and serum cholesterol and triglycerides
- Protects and improves the function of the gastrointestinal tract

Main Effect(s) on Growth		
Microbial Strain	**Fresh**	**Boiled**
Bacillus cereus *Bacillus subtilis* *Candida albicans*	Stimulation in most cases	Stimulation in most cases
Clostridium tetani *Clostridium sporogenes*	Complete inhibition in most cases	Partial or complete inhibition in most cases
Streptococcus pyogenes	Inhibition of hemolytic activity (5% sheep's blood)	Inhibition of hemolytic activity (5% sheep's blood) Bird and Serrano varieties only
Enterobacter aerogenes *Enterobacter cloacae* *Escherichia coli* *Klebsiella pneumoniae* *Proteus vulgaris* *Pseudomona saeruginosa* *Salmonella typhimurium* *Serratia marcescens* *Staphylococcus aureus* *Staphylococcus epidermidis*	No effect or not tested	No effect or not tested

Note: This table contains data for fruits of *Capsicum annuum* varieties only (Bird, Green Bell, Jalapeño, Red Chile, Serrano). For data on other capsicum species tested, please refer to the original research.

Table 7.6
Growth inhibiting effects of capsicum fruit extracts on various microbial strains.[58]

7.6.1 Contraindications

• Pregnancy and lactation: Likely safe when used in FDA-approved nonprescription topical products. Possibly unsafe when ingested orally during lactation (Dermatitis in breast-fed infants has been reported when the mothers' food was heavily spiced with red pepper). Insufficient reliable information exists on safety when used orally in amounts larger than those typically found in food; Avoid using unless under the strict supervision of a qualified healthcare practitioner.[141]

• Contraindicated with pepper, celery, mugwort and birch pollen allergies.[142,182]

• Avoid contact with injured or open skin and mucous membranes.[141]

7.6.2 Side Effects

• In rare cases, skin hypersensitivity reaction may occur (urticaria).[141]

• Capsaicin is extremely irritating to mucous membranes, even in very low concentrations.

7.6.3 Possible Interactions with Drugs

• Capsicum may interfere with activity of monoamine oxidase inhibitors by increasing catecholamine secretion.[141,158,362]

• Theoretically, capsicum may increase the effects and adverse effects of antiplatelet drugs, such as warfarin.[121,141]

• Topically applied capsaicin may contribute to the cough reflex in patients using ACE inhibitor drugs.[141]

• Theoretically, concomitant use with barbiturates and sedative drugs can cause additive effects and side effects.[141]

• Theoretically, capsicum can increase hepatic metabolism of drugs by increasing glucose-6-phosphate dehydrogenase and adipose lipase activity.[23,141]

• Ingested capsicum may reduce aspirin bioavailability.[62]

• Capsaicin may enhance absorption of theophylline.[32,141]

Note: If capsicum is applied topically, avoid additional heat application.

7.6.4 Possible Interactions with Herbs and other Dietary Supplements

- Concomitant use with herbs that have coumarin constituents or affect platelet aggregation may increase the risk of bleeding in some people.[141,354]
- Concomitant use with herbs that have sedative properties may enhance therapeutic and adverse effects.[141]

7.6.5 Possible Interactions with Lab Tests

- Urine odor: Fenugreek can cause a maple syrup odor in urine, not to be confused with "maple syrup urine" disease.[141]
- Blood glucose: Fenugreek can lower blood glucose and blood glucose test results.[141]

7.6.6 Possible Interactions with Diseases or Conditions

- Fenugreek allergy: Avoid using.
- Kidney stones: Fenugreek may decrease calcium oxalate deposition in the kidneys, reducing the risk of kidney stone formation.
- Diabetes: Fenugreek can affect blood sugar levels that should be monitored closely by diabetics.

7.6.7 Typical Dosage

- **Oral:** Dosage can range significantly and is primarily dependent upon heat units and therapeutic intention. In general: fruit, 30-120 mg 3 times daily; Capsicum tincture, 0.3-1 mL 3 times daily. Oleoresin, 0.6-2 mg 3 times daily.[141]

- **Topical:** OTC capsicum cream is applied to affected areas a maximum of 3-4 times daily for at least 3 days. Remove using dilute vinegar solution as capsaicin is not water soluble. Wash hands after application.[141]

Note: Topically applied cayenne has been shown to cause reversible sensory nerve cell degeneration.[240]

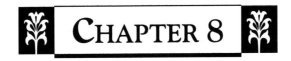

CHAPTER 8

FENUGREEK

Trigonella foenum-graecum

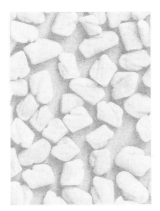

8

FENUGREEK

Trigonella foenum-graecum

8.1 Description and Medical History

Fenugreek is native to the Mediterranean region, the Ukraine, India, and China and it is widely cultivated in these regions. The fenugreek seed that is used pharmacologically comes exclusively from cultivated plants originating mainly in India, Morocco, China, and Turkey.[88]

Fenugreek is approved by the Commission E, internally to stimulate appetite and externally as a poultice for local inflammation.[30] There is growing evidence that it has a hypoglycemic effect that may function to normalize metabolism and lower blood sugar in diabetics. In addition, it has antioxidant and hypocholesterolemic actions in the body, hence its use in the treatment of atherosclerosis and elevated serum cholesterol and triglycerides levels. It has been used for numerous intestinal disorders including dyspepsia, gastritis, and constipation.[141]

Traditionally, fenugreek has been taken to reduce fever, promote lactation, and treat mouth ulcers, boils, bronchitis, tuberculosis, chronic coughs, chapped lips, and cancer.[141]

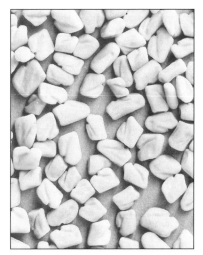

Figure 8.1
*Trigonella foenum-graecum
(fenugreek) seeds*

8.2 Known Medicinal Constituents

• Complex carbohydrates and fiber (25-45%) and protein (25-30%; rich in lysine and tryptophan but low in sulfur-containing amino acids)[88]

• Proteinase inhibitors acting on human trypsin and chymotrypsin[88]

• Steroid saponins: *trigofoenosides A-G (bitter), aglycones, including diosgenin, yamogenin, gitogenin, smilagenin, tigogenin, yuccagenin*[88]

• Flavonoids: *isoorientin (and arabinoside), isovitexin, orientin (and arabinoside), saponaretin, vicenin-1, vicenin-2, and vitexin*[88]

• Novel amino acid 4-hydroxyisoleucine (possibly involved in hypoglycemic activity)[88]

• Sterols and sterol esters[88]

8.3 Indications for Use

• Internal: Loss of appetite, anorexia, dyspepsia, gastritis, and convalescence[30]

• External (poultice): furunculosis, myalgia, lymphadenitis, gout, eczema, wounds, and leg ulcers[30]

• Hyperglycemia, non-insulin dependent and insulin dependent diabetes

• Hyperlipidemia

• Lactation difficulties

8.4 Mechanisms of Action

• Hypoglycemic activity: Fenugreek affects gastrointestinal transit time, slowing glucose absorption.[141,284]

• The amino acid constituent 4-hyrdoxyisoleucine appears to directly stimulate insulin secretion by the pancreas in a glucose-dependent manner.[34,35,141,284] In healthy people, the whole seed extract, gum isolate, cooked seed, and the constituent, trigonelline show hypoglycemic activity.[141,237]

• Non-insulin dependent diabetes: Ingestion of the extracted seeds improves plasma glucose and insulin response.[237]

• Insulin dependent diabetes: Ingestion of the seed powder reduces plasma glucose, glycosuria, and the daily insulin requirement.[237]

• Anorexia induced in rats using adrenergic agonist d-fenfluramine was not significantly prevented by fenugreek, suggesting its hypoglycemic activity is not adrenergic in nature.[255]

• Steroid saponins are thought to mediate fenugreek's potentiation of appetite.[256] They also mediate the cholesterol-lowering activity of fenugreek by inhibiting absorption of bile acids taurocholate and deoxycholate in a dose-dependent manner.[311]

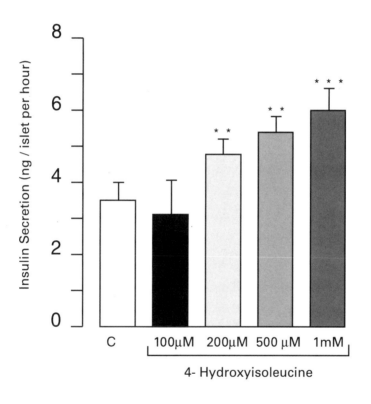

Figure 8.2
Effects of 4-hydroxyisoleucine on insulin release from isolated rat islets in the presence of 8.3 mmol/L glucose (supranormal). $*p < 0.01$; $**p < 0.001$; *Adapted from Sauvaire et al.*[284]

8.5 Research

8.5.1 Fenugreek, Blood Sugar, and Cholesterol

S auvaire et al[284] extracted and purified 4-hydroxyisoleucine, an insulinotropic agent, from fenugreek seeds. The novel amino acid increased glucose-induced insulin secretion in a dose-dependent manner by acting directly on isolated rat and human islets of Langerhans (Figure 8.2).

An interesting characteristic of 4-hydroxyisoleucine is that it only appears to be active in the presence of supranormal glucose concentrations (6.6-16.7 mmol/L). At low (3 mmol/L) and basal (5 mmol/L) concentrations of glucose, the amino acid does not stimulate insulin secretion.[284] Although the mechanism is not known, this characteristic suggests that there is a low risk for the isolated substance to cause hypoglycemia in normoglycemic individuals. However, this cannot be said conclusively for the fenugreek whole herb. It should also be noted that this study was

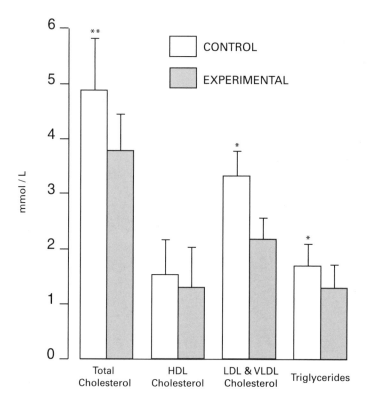

Figure 8.3
Effect of fenugreek seeds on serum lipid profile of Type I diabetics.[294] *p<0.01; **p<0.001

performed *in vitro* on isolated tissues, so it is not known if the amino acid would have the same function *in vivo*. In light of the fact that fenugreek seeds are known to have antidiabetic properties in traditional medicine, this study lends support to a clinical application of the herb in non-insulin dependent (Type II) diabetes.

Additional studies support the hypoglycemic activity of fenugreek. Fenugreek seed powder given alone or in conjunction with vanadate lowered blood sugar and increased the growth rate of chemically diabetic rats almost to control levels.[113] Because chemically-induced diabetes destroys insulin secreting cells, it seem unlikely that fenugreek acts by potentiating insulin secretion in this model. Fenugreek treatment also significantly lowered liver and kidney glucose-6-phosphate and fructose-1,6-bisphosphate levels. The combination of fenugreek and vanadate was more effective than administered insulin in restoring these parameters and fenugreek also attenuated vanadium toxicity.

In human subjects with Type I (insulin-dependent) diabetes, fenugreek seed significantly decreased fasting blood sugar and improved oral glucose tolerance test results.[294] In addition, a 54% decrease in 24-hour urinary glucose excretion was observed. Serum total, LDL, and VLDL cholesterol, and triglycerides were decreased while HDL cholesterol remained unchanged (Figure 8.3). Again, fenugreek cannot be acting as an insulinotropic agent in Type I diabetes, as a lack of insulin secreting cells is indicated in this form of the disease.

Nonetheless, these results suggest that fenugreek may be quite useful in balancing serum glucose and lipids in humans, especially with respect to the diabetic condition.

8.5.2 Antioxidant Activity of Fenugreek

Fenugreek has been shown to significantly improve blood levels of glutathione and β-carotene (antioxidants) in normal and alloxan diabetic rats.[266] Conversely, fenugreek decreased α-tocopherol levels and had no effect on ascorbic acid levels. Chemically induced diabetes in animals causes a disruption in free radical metabolism, which is normalized by supplementation with fenugreek in the diet. This study suggests that fenugreek may potentiate Phase II detoxification mechanisms.

8.6 Overview

These clinical results coupled with the results of earlier trials strongly suggest that **fenugreek:**

- Reduces blood glucose levels
- Normalizes free radical metabolism in diabetic animals

8.6.1 Contraindications

- Fenugreek allergy[141]
- Do not use during pregnancy. Fenugreek has potential oxytocic and uterine stimulant activity.[237]

8.6.2 Side Effects

- Skin sensitization is possible with repeated external use of the drug.[88,141]
- May cause oxytocic and uterine stimulant activity. Avoid using during pregnancy.[141]

8.6.3 Possible Interactions with Drugs

- Insulin/hypoglycemic drugs: Fenugreek has hypoglycemic activity and therefore has the potential to interact with hypoglycemic drugs and insulin resulting in an exaggerated hypoglycemia.[141]
- Anticoagulants: Theoretically, may potentiate anticoagulant drug activity and increase the risk of bleeding.[141]
- Hormone therapy: Theoretically, fenugreek may interfere with hormone therapy.[141]
- Monoamine oxidase inhibitors (MAOIs): Fenugreek may potentiate MAOI drug activity.[141]
- Corticosteroids: Theoretically, fenugreek may reduce corticosteroid drug activity.[141]
- All drugs: Fenugreek's high mucilage content may decrease or delay the absorption of oral drugs.[141]

8.6.4 Possible Interactions with Herbs and other Dietary Supplements

- Insufficient reliable information available.

8.6.5 Possible Interactions with Lab Tests

• Urine odor: Fenugreek can cause a maple syrup odor in urine, not to be confused with "maple syrup urine" disease.[141]

• Blood glucose: Fenugreek can lower blood glucose and blood glucose test results.[141]

8.6.6 Possible Interactions with Diseases or Conditions

• Fenugreek allergy: Avoid using.

• Kidney stones: Fenugreek may decrease calcium oxalate deposition in the kidneys, reducing the risk of kidney stone formation.

• Diabetes: Fenugreek can affect blood sugar levels that should be monitored closely by diabetics.

8.6.7 Typical Dosage

• **Oral:** In combination with other synergistic detoxifying herbs, 100 to 500 mg per day. When used alone, 1-2 grams of seed or equivalent three times daily or one cup of the tea (500 mg seed in 150 mL cold water for three hours, strained) several times a day. Do not exceed six grams of seed per day to avoid side effects.[141]

• **Topical:** (poultice): 50 grams of powdered seed in 0.25-1 L of hot water to form a paste.[141]

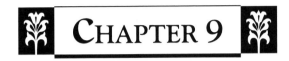
JUNIPER BERRIES

Juniperus communis

9

JUNIPER BERRIES

Juniperus communis

9.1 Description and Medical History

Juniper grows in temperate regions of the northern hemisphere, and has a natural affinity for moorlands, heaths, and chalk downs. A member of the Cupressaceae (Coniferae) family, the juniper plant produces female berries, more closely related to pine cones than to actual berries. The berries take two to three years to ripen, such that the ripe (blue) and unripe (green) berries may be found on the same tree.

Traditional uses for juniper include the treatment of cancer,[186] intestinal worms, gastrointestinal infections, snakebites, flatulence, and colic.[237] Commission E approves juniper dried fruit preparations or oil extracts to relieve dyspepsia.[30]

The popular non-medicinal use of juniper berries is for the preparation of gin and as a flavoring agent in foods and beverages. The oil is also used for its fragrant components in the manufacture of soaps and cosmetics.

Note: Completed research studies on the mechanisms of action and indications for use of juniper berries are primarily the results of tests on laboratory animals, although there is a marked interest in the scientific community for completing human studies to further validate the results of the animal studies.

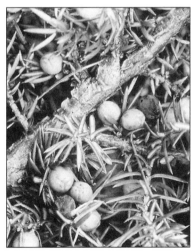

Figure 9.1
Juniperus communis (Juniper Berries)

9.2 Known Medicinal Constituents

- Antitumor agent: *podophyllotoxin*
- Bitter principle: *juniperin*
- Catechins
- Diterpene acids
- Fatty acids
- Flavonoid glycosides
- Invert sugar
- Lignans: *Desoxypodophyllotoxin*
- Organic Acids
- Proanthocyanidins
- Resin
- Volatile oils, chiefly monoterpenes: α-*pinene*, β-*pinene* , β-*myrcene*, β-*caryophylene*, *limonene*, *cadinene*, *elemene eposydihydrocaryophyllene*, β-*elemem-7-α-ol*, *terpinene-4-ol*, *sabinene*, *thujone*, *camphor*, *terpinyl acetate*, *and limonene*
- Sterols
- Tannins

9.3 Indications for Use

- Antiseptic[30,186]
- Bladder and kidney disease[186,237]
- Cystitis/infections of the urethra, bladder, and ureter[186]
- Detoxification[76,144,338]
- Diabetes-*specifically, symptoms of hyperglycemia, loss of body weight, and polydipsia.*[282,319]In a contradictory statement, the European Scientific Cooperative on Phytotherapy advises that juniper berry may increase glucose levels in diabetics.[82]
- Dyspepsia[30,339]
- Edema
- Fungal infection[112]
- Gastrointestinal symptoms: Heartburn; Bloating; Loss of appetite[112]
- Hepatic reperfusion injuries[144]
- Inflammation
- Rheumatism[339]

- Stones (Kidney and Bladder)[112]
- Tumor progression[186,216]

9.4 Mechanisms of Action

- Supports detoxification of endotoxins by blunting increases in intracellular calcium and release of prostaglandin E2 (PGE2) by cultured Kupffer cells[144]
- Supports detoxification mechanisms by improving rate of bile flow[144]
- Aquaretic effects that increase the amount of water loss through urinary excretion with no impact on electrolyte excretion[76,271]
- Terpinene-4-ol increases glomerular filtration rate with speculation that it can also irritate the kidneys, although this may not be the case with the use of whole dried berries[208]
- Volatile oils prevent antispasmodic effects in smooth muscle[186]
- Desoxypodophyllotoxin and amentoflavone may inhibit the cytotoxic actions of herpes simplex virus type 1 and exhibit general antiviral actions[30,201]
- Fungicidal against *Pennicillium notatum*
- Fatty acid components inhibit activation of Kupffer cells, reducing vasoactive eicosanoid release and improving hepatic microcirculation in livers undergoing oxidative stress.[144]
- Diaphoretic
- Encourages glucose homeostasis by reducing level of hyperglycemia during development of diabetes and reducing polydipsia and rate of weight loss associated with shifts in blood glucose levels and associated pancreatic insufficiency.[319]
- Gastrointestinal antiseptic[186]

9.5 Research

9.5.1 Juniper Berries and Liver Function

Jones et al[144] investigated the effects of juniper berry oil on hepatic reperfusion injury in rats. Juniper berry oil is rich in 5,11,14-eicosatrienic acid, a polyunsaturated fatty acid that is markedly similar to that found in dietary fish oil. However, juniper oil is less prone to the damaging effects of lipid peroxidation. Given that dietary fish oil has been shown to reduce the effects of reperfusion injury in the liver, the researchers sought to investigate if a similar effect could be found with the use of juniper berry oil.

Compared with fish oil and corn oil, juniper berry oil showed promising therapeutic effects in preventing lactate dehydrogenase (LDH) release and malondialdehyde (an end-product of lipid peroxidation) production, while also improving the rate of bile flow under oxidative stress. Juniper berry oil also reduced cell death in select regions of the liver by 75% and improved hepatic circulation, as evidenced by Trypan Blue distribution time, an indicator of hepatic microcirculation. Table 9.1 highlights the results of this study.

9.6 Overview

These clinical results coupled with the results of earlier trials strongly suggest that the **juniper berry:**

- Improves liver function
- Improves kidney function
- Improves hepatic microcirculation
- Increases bile flow rate

	Corn Oil	Fish Oil	Juniper Berry Oil
Peak LDH release during reflow (U/g/h)	44	32	21
Max MDA value: end-product of lipid peroxidation (nmol/g/h)	62	43	34
Bile Flow Rate (µL/g/h)	25	36	38
Trypan blue distribution time (% reduction- correlates to improved hepatic microcirculation)	Control	25%	50%
Rate of entry/Rate of outflow of flourescein-dextran (reflects hepatic microcirculation)	N/A	1.8- fold increase/ 4.4- fold increase	2.6-fold increase/ 4.3-fold increase

Table 9.1

Effect of Juniperus communis constituents on hepatic damage, hepatic microcirculation, and bile flow[144]

- Inhibits activation of Kupffer cells
- Decreases lactate dehydrogenase (LDH) release under oxidative stress on the liver
- Decreases lipid peroxidation following hepatic reperfusion injury
- Increases glomerular filtration rate
- Increases water loss without affecting electrolyte balance
- Decreases perineal pain
- Decreases nocturnal (nighttime) frequency
- Increases urinary flow rate
- Prevents infections due to residual urine
- Reduces residual urine
- Improves quality of life for BPH patients

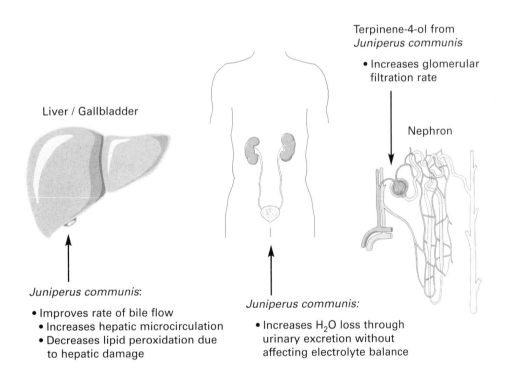

Terpinene-4-ol from
Juniperus communis

- Increases glomerular filtration rate

Nephron

Liver / Gallbladder

Juniperus communis:

- Improves rate of bile flow
  - Increases hepatic microcirculation
  - Decreases lipid peroxidation due to hepatic damage

Juniperus communis:

- Increases H_2O loss through urinary excretion without affecting electrolyte balance

Figure 9.2
Select mechanisms of action of juniper berry (Juniperus communis)

9.6.1 Contraindications

Note: Most contraindications for *Juniperus communis* refer to the prolonged use of the volatile oil extract of the berries. However, use of whole fresh and dried berries can be prescribed safely in most cases, with the exception of acute renal inflammation, where care must be exercised.

• Pregnancy: Abortifacient, increases uterine tone, interferes with fertility and implantation. Avoid use.[100]
• Lactation: Insufficient data. Avoid use.
• Active inflammation of any organ
• History of renal conditions
• Inflammatory kidney disease
• Kidney infection
• Infectious or inflammatory gastrointestinal conditions

9.6.2 Side Effects

• Side effects are only relevant with the use of excessive amounts of juniper berry oil and not with the use of whole fresh or dried berries. Overdose symptoms include kidney pain, tachycardia, hypertension, convulsions, metorrhagia, abortion, diuresis, albuminuria, and hematuria.[237]

9.6.3 Possible Interactions with Drugs

• Theoretically may interfere with diuretic therapy.[237,271]
• Diabetes: Theoretically may potentiate effects of diabetic therapy.[237]

9.6.4 Possible Interactions with Herbs and other Dietary Supplements

• None known

9.6.5 Possible Interactions with Lab Tests

• Urine Tests: Juniper berry can interfere with urine assays and cause urine discoloration (purple).[237]

9.6.6 Possible Interactions with Diseases or Conditions

- Do not use for more than 4 to 6 weeks in successive duration at a dose of over 3 grams of dried berries per day.
- Diabetes: Monitor blood glucose level closely due to potential hypoglycemic affect.[112,237, 319]
- Seizure Disorders: Theoretically may exacerbate condition.
- Cardiac insufficiency[112]
- Hypertonia[112]
- Fever[112]
- Acute skin disease[112]
- Large skin wounds[112]

9.6.7 Typical Dosage

- **Dried berry:** In combination with other synergistic detoxifying herbs, 1 to 3 grams per day. Do not exceed 10 grams per day.

- **Tincture:** (1:5 in 45% ethanol): 1-2 mL, t.i.d.

- **Liquid Extract:** (1:1 in 25% ethanol): 2-4 mL, t.i.d.

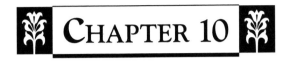

CHAPTER 10

GREATER CELANDINE

Chelidonium majus

10

-->>|*|<<--

GREATER CELANDINE

Chelidonium majus

10.1 Description and Medical History

Celandine is found in Europe and Asia in temperate and subarctic regions. It has yellow flowers and a fruit that is pod-like with many seeds. Celandine contains a dark-yellow latex sap that is fragrant.[88] The herb is hot and bitter to the taste due to its high alkaloid content.

Celandine is collected in the spring during the flowering season and the medicinal flowers and aerial parts are usually dried under high temperature.[88] The root is collected in the late summer and early fall.

Celandine herb is approved by the Commission E for liver and gallbladder complaints. It is said to be effective for treating cholecystitis, cholelithiasis, jaundice, gastroenteritis, and various liver and gall bladder complaints. However, these uses are not clinically proven.[88] Celandine has also been used for the treatment of intestinal polyps and breast lumps. In Chinese medicine it is used for a variety of ailments, including jaundice and stomach carcinomas.

Celandine root is used in folk medicine for toothache (chewed) and tooth extraction (powder). In homeopathic medicine it is used to treat gallstones and chronic disorders of the hepatobiliary system, rheumatism, and inflammation of the lungs and pleura.[88]

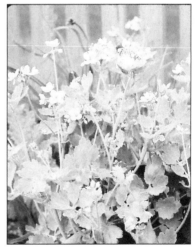

Figure 10.1
Chelidonium majus
(Greater Celandine)

10.2 Known Medicinal Constituents

- Isoquinoline alkaloids: *Protoberberine, benzophenanthridine, and protopine types. Coptisine is* the main protoberberine alkaloid. Also *berberine, chelidonine, sanguinarine, chelerythrine, protopine, and cryptopine.*[88]
- Caffeic acid and derivatives[88]

10.3 Indications for Use

- Spastic discomfort of bile ducts and gastrointestinal pain[141]
- Liver and gall bladder complaints, gout[141]
- Gallstones[78]
- Loss of appetite
- Stomach cancer, intestinal polyps, breast lumps
- Angina, arteriosclerosis, hypertension
- Topically: Warts, blisters, scabies, tooth pain
- Fungal infections (*Fusarium spp.*)[205]

10.4 Mechanisms of Action

- The isoquinoline alkaloids in greater celandine (0.1-1%) are reported to have antispasmodic and weak central analgesic activity.[124, 141]

- Celandine improves liver function mainly by increasing bile acid independent flow in the liver.[341] It has demonstrated hepatoprotective actions in animals.[141]

- A semisynthetic alkaloid derived from greater celandine, Ukrain, shows antimitotic and cytotoxic activity *in vitro*[250] Preliminary studies show that Ukrain inhibits the growth of cancer cell lines. In addition, it was shown to shrink lesions and prevent new growth in two AIDS patients with Kaposi's sarcoma.[355] It was also shown to improve immunohaematological status in these patients by increasing total leukocytes, T-lymphocytes, and T-suppressor cell numbers. In one case T-helper lymphocytes were also increased. Brain tumor growth was inhibited in a case study[312] by a presumptive immunostimulatory mechanism.[242,306,375]

10.5 Research

10.5.1 Celandine and Liver Function

In isolated perfused rat liver, greater celandine significantly increased bile-acid-independent flow (choleresis) such that the amount of bile was almost doubled 40 minutes after administration as compared with control (Figure 10.2).[341] Additionally, when administration of the extract was stopped, bile flow declined immediately, reaching pretreatment levels within 30 minutes. This result suggests that celandine is a valuable herb for rapid restoration of sluggish bile flow.

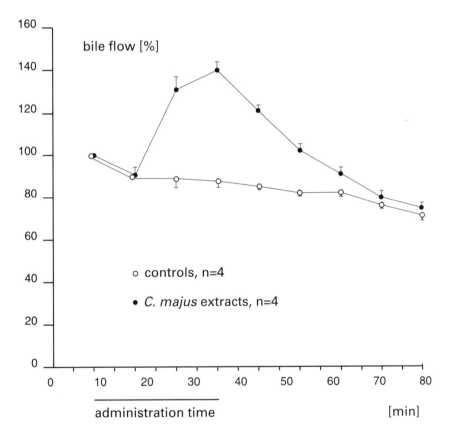

Figure 10.2
Increased bile flow in % after administration of total extract of C. majus *(10 mg/mL/min).*
AUC was 916.1±26.5 for the experimental group vs. 740.3±21.7 for the control group (p<0.025).[341]

Although celandine effectively increased bile flow, bile acid production was not altered by the extract (Figure 10.3). This effect may reduce the risk of gallstone formation.

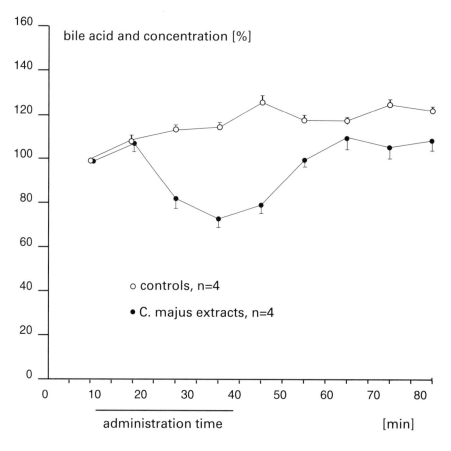

Figure 10.3
Decreased bile acid concentration in % after administration of total extract of C. majus (10 mg/mL/min). AUC was 897.5±47.2 for the experimental group vs. 1058.6±16.6 for the control group (p<0.025).[341]

10.5.2 Celandine and Cancer

Celandine and two other herbs used medicinally in China were examined for their anticancer effects in human subjects with advanced stage esophageal squamous cell carcinom.[375] Extracts of the herbs alone or in conjunction with endoxan (cyclophosphamide) were administered regularly to cancer patients for two weeks prior to surgery. A control group received no pretreatment. Esophageal tissues and regional lymph nodes were surgically removed and quantitatively examined for the following:

• Degree of degenerative changes in cancer parenchyma, especially in the marginal areas of infiltration

• Stromal lymphoid cell responses around the carcinomas

• Morphology of the regional lymph nodes (degree of follicular hyperplasia and sinus histiocytosis)

Tables 10.1 and 10.2 show the results. Cancer cell degeneration was slight to negligible in the control group but significant in both the celandine and celandine+endoxan groups (Table 10.1).

Group	Treatment (N)	Agent used	Cancer cell degeneration: # of cases (%)				
			None	Slight	Moderate	Severe	Total
A	Chinese herbs only[98]	Menispernum dehuricum DC**	9(18.0)	22(44.0)	14(28.0)	5(10.0)	50(100)
		Chelidonium majus L**	5(16.7)	9(30.0)	13(43.3)	3(10.0)	30(100)
		Camptothecinum	4(22.2)	7(38.9)	5(27.8)	2(11.1)	18(100)
B	Chinese herbs + endoxan[42]	*Chelidonium majus* L + endoxan*	3(17.6)	8(47.1)	3(17.6)	3(17.6)	17(100)
		Camptothecinum + endoxan	9(36.0)	8(32.0)	6(24.0)	2(8.0)	25(100)
C	Control[100]	None	50(50.0)	35(35.0)	12(12.0)	3(3.0)	100(100)

*$p<0.05$ **$p<0.01$

Table 10.1

Degree of cancer cell degeneration after treatment with celandine and other herbs with or without endoxan.[375]

Group	Treatment (N)	Agent used	Cancer cell degeneration: # of cases (%)				
			None	Slight	Moderate	Severe	Total
A	Chinese herbs only[98]	Menispernum dehuricum DC**	0(0)	15(30.0)	19(38.0)	16(32.0)	50(100)
		Chelidonium majus L*	0(0)	12(40.0)	11(36.7)	7(23.3)	30(100)
		Camptothecinum**	1(5.6)	8(44.4)	7(38.9)	2(11.1)	18(100)
B	Chinese herbs + endoxan[42]	*Chelidonium majus* L + endoxan	2(11.8)	5(29.4)	9(52.9)	1(5.9)	17(100)
		Camptothecinum + endoxan	4(16.0)	9(36.0)	12(48.0)	0(0)	25(100)
C	Control[100]	None	12(12.0)	51(51.0)	30(30.0)	7(7.0)	100(100)

*$p<0.05$ **$p<0.01$

Table 10.2

Grade of lymphoid cell response in peripheral areas of invading cancer cells after treatment with celandine and other herbs with or without endoxan.[375]

Severe cancer cell degeneration was greatest in the celandine+endoxan group. However, celandine alone showed the greatest combined percentage of severe and moderate cancer cell degeneration. Celandine alone also significantly improved the grade of lymphoid cell response in peripheral areas of invading cancer cells although in conjunction with endoxan it was not significant (Table 10.2).

10.6 Overview

These clinical results coupled with the results of earlier trials strongly suggest that **Celandine:**

- Functions as a chemoprotective agent
- Improves liver function
- Improves bile flow
- Improves intestinal function

10.6.1 Contraindications

- Pregnancy: Berberine content may stimulate uterine contractions; Do not use during pregnancy.
- Aerial parts contraindicated in hepatitis/liver disease (see *Side Effects*).

10.6.2 Side Effects

- A small number of putative cases of celandine-induced acute hepatitis have been reported; Celandine containing products should not be used for more than one month at a time.[27]

10.6.3 Possible Interactions with Drugs

- Aerial parts may affect drugs used for treatment of glaucoma[141]

10.6.4 Possible Interactions with Herbs and other Dietary Supplements

• Insufficient reliable information available

10.6.5 Possible Interactions with Lab Tests

• Liver function tests: Possibility of increased liver enzymes in serum

10.6.6 Possible Interactions with Diseases or Conditions

• Celandine may exacerbate bile tract obstruction[141]
• Celandine may affect glaucoma treatment

10.6.7 Typical Dosage

Aerial parts:
• Oral: 2-6 grams of the dried, above-ground parts or tea (2-6 grams in 150 mL boiling water for 5-10 minutes, strained) three times daily. Liquid extract (1:1 in 25% ethanol): 2-6 mL three times daily. Tincture (1:5 in 45% ethanol): 2-8 mL three times daily.

Root/rhizome:
• Standard dose is 500 mg.
• Drug is light-sensitive. Store away from light.

In combination with other synergistic detoxifying herbs, 600 to 1200 mg of the whole herb per day.

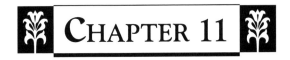

CHAPTER 11

FRINGE TREE

Chionanthus

11

⇒⟫❂⟨⇐

FRINGE TREE

Chionanthus

11.1 Description and Medical History

Fringe tree is a deciduous shrub or tree that may grow up to 10 meters in height. The tree bears large white flowers on long peduncles and the bark of fringe tree is so dense that it sinks in water, unlike most other barks. The root and the bark are both used medicinally, primarily for liver and gall bladder complaints.[88]

Fringe tree is odorless but very bitter to the taste.[141] The hepatoprotective use of the root is reported frequently in homeopathic and folk medicine.[88]

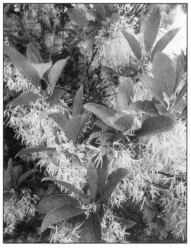

Figure 11.1
Chionanthus (Fringe Tree)

11.2 Known Medicinal Constituents

- Lignan glycosides: *Phillyrin (chioanthine)*
- Saponins

11.3 Indications for Use

- Clinical Purification
- Liver and gall bladder disorders, including gallstones[141]

11.4 Mechanisms of Action

- The saponins in fringe tree are said to have hepatic, cholagogue, diuretic, and tonic effects.[88]

11.5 Overview

Fringe tree may be beneficial in:

- Supporting the liver detoxification process
- Protecting the liver from damage

11.5.1 Contraindications

- None known
- Pregnancy and lactation: Insufficient information; avoid using

11.5.2 Side Effects

- None known

11.5.3 Possible Interactions with Drugs

- None known

11.5.4 Possible Interactions with Herbs and other Dietary Supplements

- None known

11.5.5 Possible Interactions with Lab Tests

- None known

11.5.6 Possible Interactions with Diseases or Conditions

- None known

11.5.7 Typical Dosage

- Fringe tree is generally used as a liquid extract, although dried root powder is frequently used in combination with other synergistic liver detoxifying herbs in amounts not to exceed 1 gram per day.

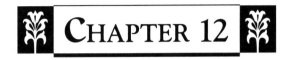

CHAPTER 12

MILK THISTLE

Silybum marianum

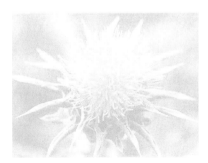

12

⤞⤏✳⤌⤝

MILK THISTLE

Silybum marianum

12.1 Description and Medical History

Milk thistle is a perennial herb indigenous to Europe and naturalized in North America.[77] It is often found growing in rocky, waste places. Milk thistle gets its name from the milky sap that is exuded by the leaves when they are broken or torn.[141]

It is the ripe seeds of milk thistle that are medicinally active.[88] The Commission E has approved milk thistle seed for treatment of dyspeptic, liver, and gall bladder complaints.[88] Silymarin, the active component in milk thistle, is a mixture of several active flavonoids, including silibinin. It is used successfully in the clinical treatment of chronic hepatopathies involving degenerative necrosis and functional impairment.[233,343]

There is evidence to suggest several mechanisms of protection offered by silymarin. It appears to stabilize cell membranes, scavenge low molecular weight free radicals, and maintain the levels of antioxidant molecules in cells under oxidative stress.[343] Silymarin appears to have an

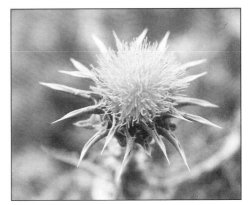

Figure 12.1
Silybum marianum (Milk Thistle) Seeds

affinity for liver and intestinal tissues in humans and rats, as it is found to be most prevalent in those tissues after ingestion. 80% of ingested silymarin and its metabolites are excreted as glucuronide conjugates by the biliary tract. It is believed that the flavonoid initiates a cyclic entero-hepatic circulation when gut flora break down the conjugates and free silymarin for reabsorption.[192,342] Not surprisingly, silymarin is most effective in elevating glutathione levels in the liver, stomach, and intestine.

12.2 Known Medicinal Constituents

- Silymarin (flavonolignan mixture, 1.5-3.0%): silybin A, silybin B (mixture of A and B is called silibinin), isosilybin A, isosilybin B, silychristin, and silydianin chiefly[88]
- Flavonoids: apigenin, chrysoeriol, eriodictyol, naringenin, quercetin, and taxifolin[88]
- Fatty oils (20-30%)

12.3 Indications for Use

Internal
- Catarrh of the bile duct and decreased bile flow[77]
- Gallstones
- Jaundice
- Poor hepatic circulation
- Prostate cancer
- Toxic liver damage: Alcoholic liver cirrhosis, Child's A group portal hypertension, Amanita phalloides (death cap) mushroom poisoning (intravenous use of silymarin only)[141]

External
- Skin conditions: Warts, corns, epithelioma, urticaria, and eczema[77]

12.4 Possible Mechanisms of Action

- The components of silymarin appear to inhibit the entrance of toxins into the liver by blocking toxin-binding sites and altering the outer cell membrane of liver cells.[184,343] Silymarin may decrease the rate of phospholipid and cholesterol turnover in liver cell membranes.[221,233]   In addition, it increases production of glutathione, a detoxification molecule, and scavenges prooxidant free radicals.[342,343] Silymarin also stimulates RNA and DNA synthesis in the nuclei of hepatocytes by a steroid-like regulatory action, increasing ribosomal and protein synthesis and hence the ability of the liver to regenerate following toxic exposure.[88] It has been used successfully as an adjunctive treatment in death-cap mushroom poisoning, a condition in which RNA polymerase I is inhibited by α-amanitin causing the liver to degenerate rapidly.[90]

• Silymarin appears to be chemoprotective in numerous *in vitro* studies of human and animal cancer cell lines.[175,394,395,396] It appears to act via several mechanisms depending on cell type, including inhibition of :

> – Protein kinases[11,395,396]
>
> – mRNA expression and tumor necrosis factor α [394]
>
> – Carcinogen-induced hyperplasia and lipid peroxidation.[175]

• Silibinin is thought to mediate hepatoprotection via the intensely phagocytic Kupffer cells on which it acts.[88] Silibinin decreases the production of superoxide radicals, nitric oxide, and leukotrienes by these cells, thereby decreasing inflammation and reactive oxygen damage. It also mildly chelates iron, decreasing hepatic and mitochondrial glutathione oxidation induced by iron overload.[258]

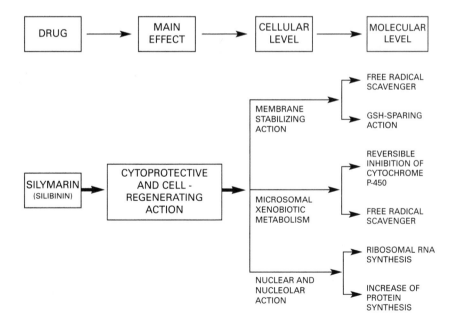

Figure 12.2
Putative main cytoprotective actions of silymarin at the cellular and molecular levels.

• Silibinin has been shown to reduce prostate-specific antigen (PSA) levels in hormone-refractory prostate carcinomas[397] and inhibit cancer cell growth by decreasing protein kinase and associated cyclin levels in the cells.

• Silymarin can decrease elevated levels of aspartate aminotransferase and alanine aminotransferase, as well as serum and conjugated bilirubin, in human patients with liver disease, correlating with normalization of liver histologic changes.[280]

12.5 Research

12.5.1 Milk Thistle and Hepatoprotection

Silymarin has been successfully used to normalize serum levels of liver enzymes in the treatment of compensated alcoholic cirrhosis in humans.[177] A thrice-daily oral ingestion of 140 mg silymarin (Legalon®) significantly lowered elevated enzyme levels to close to the normal range in cirrhosis patients. It is noteworthy that many of the subjects in this study continued to drink alcohol during the study period, although alcohol consumption was reduced.

Enzyme	Upper limit of normal range	Control group (n=20)		Silymarin group (n=20)	
		Before treatment	After treatment	Before treatment	After treatment
Bilirubin (mM/L)	20	24±6	22±8	29±6	18±7[a]
Aspartate aminotransferase (U/L)	20	58±12	52±13	55±10	28±11[c]
Alanine aminotransferase (U/L)	20	24±8	26±8	27±9	13±10[b]
g-glutamyl transferase (U/L)	25	64±12	72±12	72±13	42±11[a]

* Legalon® , a commercially available oral silymarin supplement, was used in this study.
[a] ($p<0.05$) [b] ($p<0.025$) [c] ($p<0.01$)

Table 12.1
Effect of silymarin (3x140mg silymarin daily for one month) treatment on
serum levels of liver enzymes in humans with compensated alcoholic liver cirrhosis[177]*

12.5.2 Milk Thistle and Cancer

Numerous researchers[175,394,395,396] have conducted experiments examining the effect of silymarin on *in vivo* tumorigenesis and the growth of human and animal cancer cell lines *in vitro*. The effects are quite remarkable. Silymarin was shown to possess high to complete protective activity against experimentally induced skin tumorigenesis in mice in a dose dependent manner (Figure 12.3 and Table 12.2). Topical application of silymarin prior to treatment of skin with tumor promoters, 12-O-tetradecanoylphorbol 13-acetate (TPA) and okadaic acid (OA), resulted in exceptionally high protection against tumor promotion in these mice (Data for TPA shown in Figure 12.3; Complete protection was found for OA.)

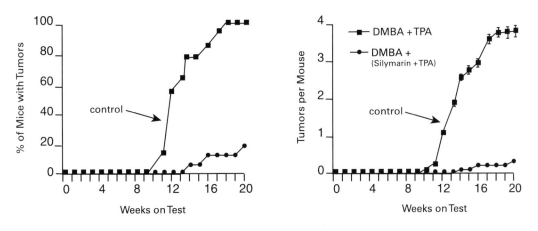

Figure 12.3
Protective effect of silymarin against tumor incidence and multiplicity during TPA-induced tumor promotion in mice. Treatments were performed twice weekly for 20 weeks. Treatment groups consisted of 20 mice each. DMBA was used as an initiating agent.[394]

Silymarin also dramatically reduced DNA synthesis in human epidermoid carcinoma A431 cells as evidenced by a reduction in [³H]-Thymidine incorporation with increasing concentrations of silymarin (Figure 12.4).

It is thought that oxidative stress largely contributes to the tumor-promoting potential of skin cancer-promoting factors, such as phorbol ester and UV radiation.[49,157,159] Reactive oxygen species produced under oxidative stress conditions attack cellular targets like DNA, proteins, and lipid membranes. Lipid peroxide products formed in these reactions can be measured spectrophotometrically and are a good indicator of the antioxidant activity of endogenously applied compounds. Lahiri-Chatterjee et al[175] added silymarin to *in vitro* cultures of epidermal microsomes from SENCAR mice, prone to development of cancer, and found a strong inhibition of lipid peroxidation by silymarin (Figure 12.5)

This result supports the hypothesis that the chemoprotective activity of silymarin is due in part to its function as an antioxidant.

The likely biochemical mechanism by which silymarin protects against skin cancer is an inhibition of tyrosine kinase activity by the epidermal growth factor receptor (EGFR) and perturbation of cell cycle progression.[11] EGFR activation is believed to be involved in development of skin malignancies. Treatment with silymarin of human epidermoid carcinoma cells A431 over-expressing EGFR resulted in almost complete inhibition of ligand-induced EGFR tyrosine kinase activity and significantly decreased downstream tyrosine phosphorylation in these cells.

No toxicity has ever been observed with silymarin and there is no known lethal dose in animals.[79]

Treatment	Total # of tumors	Total tumor volume (mm³)	Tumor volume per mouse (mm³)	Tumor volume per tumor (mm³)
DMBA + TPA	340 (0% inhibition)	17,525 (0% inhibition)	876 (0% inhibition)	51±22
DMBA + (3 mg silymarin + TPA)	83* (76% inhibition)	4,150* (76% inhibition)	207* (76% inhibition)	50±14
DMBA + (6 mg silymarin+TPA)	53* (84% inhibition)	1,066* (94% inhibition)	53* (94% inhibition)	20±4*
DMBA + (12 mg silymarin+TPA)	11* (97% inhibition)	696* (96% inhibition)	35* (96% inhibition)	63±15

* $p < 0.001$ Treatments were performed twice weekly for 20 weeks. Treatment groups consisted of 20 mice each. DMBA was used as an initiating agent.

Table 12.2
Topical application of silymarin prior to TPA-induced tumor promotion results in significant protection against increases in tumor number and size in mice. Adapted from Lahiri-Chatterjee et al (175).

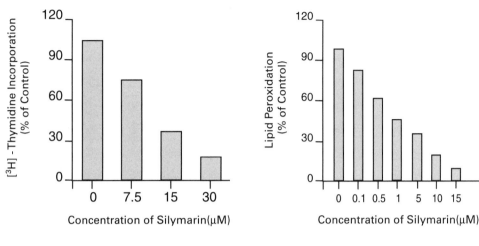

Figure 12.4

Inhibitory effect of silymarin on DNA synthesis in human epidermoid carcinoma A431 cells.[175]

Figure 12.5.

Inhibitory effect of silymarin on lipid peroxidation in SENCAR mouse epidermal microsomes under oxidative stress (Fe^{3+}).[175]

12.5.3 Milk Thistle and Cholesterol

Research by Nassuato et al[233] strongly suggests that silibinin, a primary constituent of silymarin, reduces biliary cholesterol concentration by decreasing liver cholesterol synthesis. In rats, biliary cholesterol and phospholipids were significantly reduced (60.9% and 72.9% of controls, respectively) following treatment with 100 mg silibinin per kg body weight daily for seven days. Total bile salt concentration was not significantly affected. Cholesterol excretion relative to bile flow was also reduced in silibinin-treated rats. Bile flow was unchanged between control and treated rats, suggesting biliary cholesterol reduction is due to decreased hepatic cholesterol synthesis rather than dilution by increased bile production.

In humans, oral silibinin (420 mg/day) administered to cholecystectomized patients for a month caused a significant decrease in biliary cholesterol concentration relative to controls (233; Table 12.3). All patients were on a controlled diet of 1980 kcal/day containing 60 grams of lipids during the study period. The cholesterol saturation index, a measure of the biliary lipid composition, was normalized in five of the 10 silibinin-treated patients but in only one of the nine patients receiving placebo.

Silymarin was similar to probucol, an antiatherosclerotic drug, in dose-dependently reducing cholesterol in rats.[166] Unlike probucol, however, silymarin increased HDL cholesterol and decreased liver total cholesterol, effects considered beneficial to health. In addition, silymarin partially prevented the decrease in hepatic reduced glutathione caused by feeding the rats a high-cholesterol diet, supporting its antioxidant role.

Treatment	Cholesterol (mol%)		Phospholipids (mol%)		Total Bile Salts (mol%)	
	Before	After	Before	After	Before	After
Silymarin (n=6)	10.3±4.3	5.2±1.1*	11.5±6.4	13.4±6.0	78.2±9.3	81.4±6.7
Placebo (n=9)	7.3±2.0	8.0±2.3	15.2±5.0	15.6±5.5	76.8±7.1	76.5±7.3

* $p<0.02$

Table 12.3
Biliary composition in cholecystectomized patients before and after silymarin
(420 mg/day for 30 days) or placebo treatment. Adapted from Nassuato et al.[233]

12.6 Overview

These clinical results coupled with the results of earlier trials strongly suggest that **milk thistle:**

- Protects against cancer
- Improves liver function
- Protects the liver from toxins
- Provides antioxidant protection against lipid peroxidation
- Reduces prostate-specific antigen (PSA) levels in hormone-refractory prostate carcinomas

12.6.1 Contraindications

- Allergies to the Asteraceae/Compositae plant family: ragweed, chrysanthemum, marigold, daisy, and several related herbs
- Pregnancy and lactation: Insufficient information; avoid using

12.6.2 Side Effects

- Possible mild laxative effect[141]

12.6.3 Possible Interactions with Drugs

• Concomitant use of silymarin with butyrophenones or phenothiazines (psychotropic drugs) results in reduced lipid peroxidation[248]

• Silymarin helps prevent liver damage caused by some drugs, including acetominophen, alcohol, and halothane.[141,343]

12.6.4 Possible Interactions with Herbs and other Dietary Supplements

• None known

12.6.5 Possible Interactions with Lab Tests

• Liver enzymes: Silymarin decreases elevated serum levels of transaminases and affects liver enzyme test results.[141]

12.6.6 Possible Interactions with Diseases or Conditions

• None known

12.6.7 Typical Dosage

• **Oral:** 12-15 grams of seed per day; Infusion: 3 grams of ground seed added to cold water and brought to boil, drained after 10-20 minutes, 2-3 cups daily.[88] When used as a synergistic ingredient in a liver detoxification formula, at least 200 mg of ground seed per day.

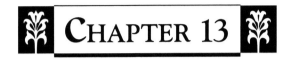

CHAPTER 13

BEET ROOT

Beta vulgaris

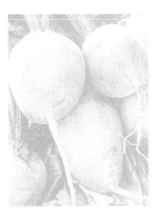

13

BEET ROOT

Beta vulgaris

13.1 Description and Medical History

Beet is a perennial indigenous to the coastal regions of Europe, North Africa, and Asia.[88] The medicinal value of beet is found in its large tuberous root, which is often deeply red in color as well as its leaves.

Beet has traditionally been used as a supportive therapy in diseases of the liver and "fatty liver." In Indian medicine it has been used to treat coughs and infections.[88] Animal studies have shown dietary beet root fiber to reduce serum and liver lipids.[22,163,185]

The main effect of beet root is antihepatotoxic. In animal tests, beet root effectively keeps fat from accumulating in the liver, probably due to the high concentration of betaine, a methyl group donor involved in the liver's transmethylation reactions.[88]

Beet fiber may improve function in the small intestine and reduce the risk of enteric infections.[39]

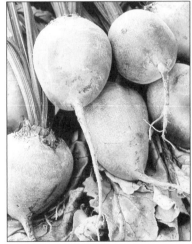

Figure 13.1
Beta vulgaris (Beet Root)

13.2 Known Medicinal Constituents

- Sugars: saccharose (up to 27% in the pressed sugar beet), oligosaccharides(refined sugar and ketose), and polysaccharides (galactans, arabans, pectin)[88]
- Fruit acids: L(-)-malic, D(+)-tartaric, oxaluric, adipic, citric, glycolic, and glutaric acids
- Amino acids: asparagine, glutamine
- Betaine (trimethylglycine)
- Triterpene saponins

13.3 Indications for Use

- Liver diseases and "fatty liver"
- Hypercholesterolemia

13.4 Mechanisms of Action

- It is not entirely clear how beet improves the function of the liver. It has been proposed that betaine, found in high quantities in beet, is responsible for its hepatoprotective function.[88,141] Betaine is a methyl donor and may facilitate methylation reactions in Phase II enzymatic detoxification in the liver.[209]

- Beet fiber significantly decreases glucose uptake from the intestine and helps to stabilize postprandial serum glucose levels in humans.[54] The beet fiber is thought to absorb and hold water and along with it dietary glucose.

13.5 Research

13.5.1 Beet and Lipid Metabolism

Sugar beet fiber fed to rats as 30% of a low fat diet for three weeks significantly decreased ileal apolipoprotein B mRNA expression that is responsible for LDL cholesterol synthesis.[207] As a possible consequence, fecal bile salt and cholesterol excretions were elevated. Beet fiber also significantly increased hepatic LDL receptor mRNA and lowered serum total and LDL cholesterol levels relative to cellulose and mushroom fiber (chitin) in rats[96] (Figures 13.2 and 13.3). The beet's demonstrated lipid lowering effect may be a result of the food's ability to increase the uptake of LDL cholesterol by the liver.

13.5.2 Beet, Cholesterol, Atherosclerosis, and Colon Cancer

Because increased serum cholesterol levels are a risk factor in colon carcinogenesis and atherosclerosis, Bobek et al[31] examined the effect of red beet fiber on the development of alimentary hypercholesterolemia and dimethylhydrazine-induced carcinogenesis in the rat colon. The researchers showed that 15% red beet fiber in a hypercholesterolemic diet (0.3% dietary cholesterol) reduced serum cholesterol and triacylglycerol levels by 30% and 40%, respectively, and increased the fraction of HDL cholesterol. Of particular interest to researchers is the significant decrease in aortic cholesterol (nearly 30%) (Table 13.1).

Red beet fiber caused a pronounced increase in the activities of superoxide dismutase, catalase, glutathione peroxidase, and glutathione-S-transferase enzymes in colon, liver, and

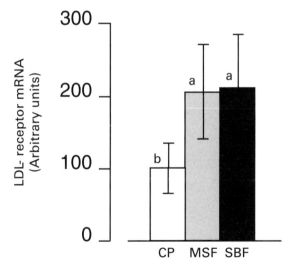

Figure 13.2

Hepatic LDL cholesterol receptor mRNA concentration in rats fed either cellulose powder (CP), mushroom fiber (MSF), or sugar beet fiber (SBF) for four weeks. Both the mushroom fiber and the sugar beet fiber groups differed significantly from the cellulose group (n=5, p<0.05).[96]

erythrocytes, supporting a hypothesis that oxidation pathways contribute to the disease state (data not shown), and illustrating that beet fiber likely promotes Phase II detoxification function in the intestine, blood, and liver. In addition, dietary red beet fiber reduced the incidence of precancerous lesions in the rat colon. Other animal studies support the finding that dietary beet fiber dose-dependently decreases serum and liver cholesterol levels.[22,163]

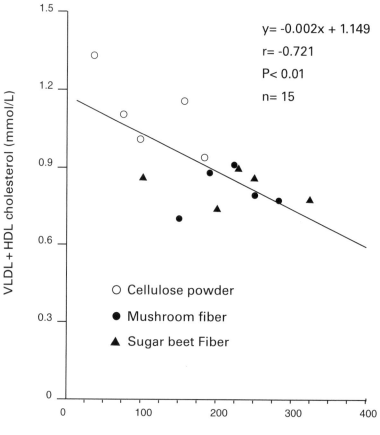

Figure 13.3
Relationship between hepatic LDL receptor mRNA level and serum VLDL+HDL+LDL cholesterol concentration in rats fed either cellulose powder (CP),mushroom fiber (MSF), or sugar beet fiber (SBF) for four weeks.[96]

Parameter	Diet		
	5% Cellulose	15% Cellulose	15% Red beet fiber
N	11	12	11
Body weight (g)	450±16	455±16	471±17
Cholesterol			
Serum (mmol/L)	9.93±0.22	9.19±0.47	6.82±0.53b,C
VLDL (mmol/L)	1.86±0.13	1.61±0.11	0.69±0.07c,C
%VLDL*	19.2±1.1	18.4±1.1	10.6±0.9c,C
LDL (mmol/L)	4.72±0.43	3.93±0.37	2.79±0.36B
%LDL*	48.5±1.9	45.1±1.6	42.7±2.0
HDL (mmol/L)	3.14±0.24	3.19±0.25	3.05±0.43
%HDL*	32.3±1.1	36.5±1.3	46.7±1.9C
Liver (mmol/kg)	511±7	496±13	523±22
Heart (mmol/kg)	10.06±0.66	9.78±0.66	8.67±0.49
Aorta (mmol/kg)	7.46±0.33	7.23±0.37	5.54±0.34b,B
Triacylglycerols			
Serum (mmol/L)	0.76±0.03	0.67±0.05	0.44±0.03c,C
Liver (mmol/L)	48.6±4.2	38.1±5.82	45.1±6.9
Heart (mmol/kg)	1.54±0.11	1.17±0.15	1.26±0.18

* Fraction of total serum cholesterol

Statistically significant against 15% cellulose diet:
a p<0.05   b p<0.01 c   p<0.001

Statistically significant against 5% cellulose diet:
A p<0.05 B p<0.01 C p<0.001

Table 13.1
*Lipids in serum, lipoproteins, and organs of rats fed a hypercholesterolemic
diet with either 5% cellulose, 15% cellulose, or 15% red beet fiber.*[31]

13.6 Overview

These clinical results coupled with the results of earlier trials strongly suggest that **beet root:**

- Has a lipid lowering effect on animals
- Promotes antioxidant activity in colon, liver, and erythrocytes, probably via improved Phase II detoxification mechanisms
- Is chemoprotective in animals

13.6.1 Contraindications

- Kidney disease: Ingestion of large quantities of beets and beet powder may worsen kidney disease.[141]

Note: At the levels found in food and designated therapeutic dosages, this danger is minimal.

13.6.2 Side Effects

- Very large quantities may lead to hypocalcemia and kidney damage due to the oxaluric acid content.[88]
- No health hazards or side effects have been reported with the amounts consumed in food or with proper administration of therapeutic dosages.[88]

13.6.3 Possible Interactions with Drugs

- None known

13.6.4 Possible Interactions with Herbs and other Dietary Supplements

- Insufficient reliable information available

13.6.5 Possible Interactions with Lab Tests

• None known

13.6.6 Possible Interactions with Diseases or Conditions

• May exacerbate symptoms of kidney disease.[141]

13.6.7 Typical Dosage

• Beet is taken orally as a granular powder. In combination with other synergistic detoxifying herbs, 300 mg or more per day. Alone, 1 or more grams per day.

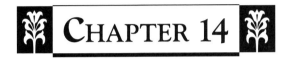

CHAPTER 14

SPANISH BLACK RADISH

Raphanus sativus niger

14

❋

SPANISH BLACK RADISH

Raphanus sativus niger

14.1 Description and Medical History

Radishes are annual or biennial plants, most likely indigenous to China and Japan, though they are now cultivated throughout the world. The medicinal part of the black radish is the root.

Radish is approved by the Commission E for treating:

• Cough and bronchitis

• Dyspeptic complaints, especially dyskinesia of the bile ducts

In folk, Chinese, and Indian medicine, the radish is used to treat coughs, gallstones, and poor digestion. It promotes bile secretion in the upper digestive tract as well as intestinal motility.[88] It is secretolytic in patients suffering from chronic bronchitis. Radish is also thought to be antimicrobial.[112]

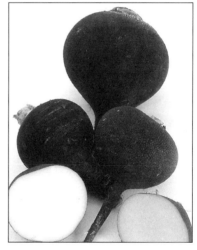

Figure 14.1
Raphanus sativus niger
(Spanish Black Radish)

14.2 Known Medicinal Constituents

- Glucosinolates in the fresh, unbruised rhizome
- Mustard oils

14.3 Indications for Use

- Clinical Purification
- Respiratory inflammation
- Dyspepsia
- Reduced bile duct motility

14.4 Possible Mechanisms of Action

- Mustard oils are thought to be responsible for the radish's choleretic, antimicrobial, and intestinal stimulatory effects.[88]
- Radishes contain defensins, molecules with antifungal activity.[81,160,247,331,332]

14.5 Research

14.5.1 Antioxidant Activity of Black Radish

Lugasi[194] examined the *in vitro* antioxidant activity of the squeezed juice from black radish. It showed strong hydrogen-donating ability, reducing power, and a copper(II)-chelating property (Tables 14.1 and 14.2, and Figure 14.2). The researchers proposed that the high level of polyphenols in the juice mediated at least some of the antioxidant activity and further showed that black radish juice had peroxide and hydroxyl radical scavenging activity as measured by luminol-dependent chemiluminometry (data not shown).

The hydrogen-donating ability is an indicator of primary chain-breaking antioxidants.[194] These antioxidants donate hydrogen to free radicals producing non-radical species and inhibiting the propagation phase of lipid oxidation.

Chelating agents play a major role in the prevention of lipid peroxidation. The decomposition of lipid hydroperoxides is catalyzed by metal ions ($Fe2+$ and $Cu2+$) and results in a rapid increase of free radicals and subsequent chain reactions.[194]

Sample	Absorbance (517 nm)	Inhibition (%)
Control	0.604±0.005	---
0.05 mL juice	0.560±0.005	7.3
0.10 mL juice	0.519±0.003	14.1
0.20 mL juice	0.447±0.001	26.0
0.50 mL juice	0.307±0.002	49.2
0.75 mL juice	0.212±0.006	64.9
1.00 mL juice	0.072±0.001	88.1

Note: All absorbance values were significantly different from control and adjacent values at $p<0.05$ probability level.

Table 14.1

Hydrogen-donating ability of black radish squeezed juice (194). Hydrogen-donating ability is expressed as reduction of 1,1-diphenyl-2-picrylhydrazyl (DPPH) radical, a pigmented molecule that absorbs at 517 nanometers.

Sample	Chelating ability (Abs485/Abs530)
Control (Cu2+)	3.22±0.05
0.1 mL juice	2.80±0.03
0.2 mL juice	2.55±0.01
0.5 mL juice	1.97±0.01
1.0 mL juice	1.65±0.02

Note: Chelating ability values were significantly different from control and adjacent values at $p<0.05$ probability level.

Table 14.2

Chelating ability of black radish squeezed juice.[194] Chelating ability is expressed as the absorbance ratio of unchelated (485 nm) to chelated (530 nm) metal ion. Thus, the sample with the lowest ratio has the highest chelating ability.

The reducing power of 1 mL of black radish juice was equivalent to 0.73 mmol ascorbic acid. Reducing power is an index of secondary antioxidant activity.[194] Secondary antioxidants inhibit the rate of lipid peroxidation by reducing transitional or end products of the lipid peroxidation process. Considering the potential damage to DNA that is caused by ascorbic acid, this research provides promising evidence for the use of a whole food, rather than an isolated fraction of the vitamin C complex, due to its safety and efficacy as an inhibitor of lipid peroxidation.

14.6 Overview

These clinical results coupled with the results of earlier trials strongly suggest that **Spanish black radish:**

- Improves bile flow
- Functions as an antioxidant

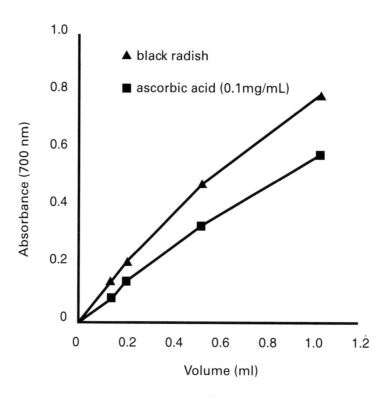

Figure 14.2
Reducing power of black radish juice relative to ascorbic acid.[194]

14.6.1 Contraindications

• Cholelithiasis: Radish is contraindicated in patients with gallstones as the choleretic effect may induce biliary colic.[112,141] *It is interesting to note that the historical use for Spanish Black Radish, the treatment of gallstones, is now considered a contraindication by modern scientists. In this case, the author questions the position stated by such authoritative figures, and suspects that future research in this area will reveal this historical truth veiled by modern science.*

14.6.2 Side Effects

• None known

14.6.3 Possible Interactions with Drugs

• None known

14.6.4 Possible Interactions with Herbs and other Dietary Supplements

• Insufficient reliable information available

14.6.5 Possible Interactions with Lab Tests

• None known

14.6.6 Possible Interactions with Diseases or Conditions

• Use with caution in patients with obstructed bile duct

14.6.7 Typical Dosage

• **Oral:** 0.5 tablespoons of the pressed root juice several times a day. 50-100 mL per day or up to 3 grams of the dried root may be taken without adverse effect. In combination with other synergistic detoxifying herbs, 300 mg or more of the dried root per day.

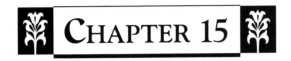

CHAPTER 15

APPLE PECTIN

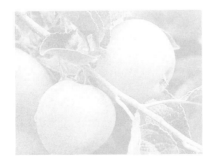

15

❖

APPLE PECTIN

15.1 Description and Medical History

Apple pectin is the soluble fiber fraction of the apple fruit. Pectin comes in liquid or dried form and the source is the solid fruit residue with 10-20% pectin in the dried mass.[88] The pectin is extracted from the dried residue at pH 1.5-3 and at temperatures ranging from 60-100°C.

Apple trees are cultivated throughout the Northern Hemisphere, occasionally growing wild. The saying, "an apple a day keeps the doctor away," has some basis in fact, as apple pectin holds preventive activity in cancer and cardiovascular disease. Preliminary evidence suggests a positive relationship between lung function and consumption of five or more apples per week.[43] An inverse association may exist between lung cancer risk and foods containing quercetin, found in high concentrations in apples.[178] Further controlled clinical human studies must be performed to confirm these results.

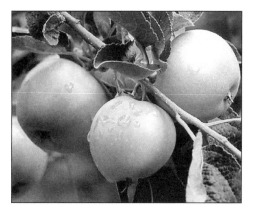

Figure 15.1
Apple tree

15.2 Known Medicinal Constituents

- Fruit acids, chiefly malic acid
- Quercetin and other flavonoids
- Pectins
- Tannins
- Vitamins, especially ascorbic acid (3-30mg / 100g)

15.3 Indications for Use

- Clinical Purification
- Impaired lung function
- Lung cancer
- Colon cancer
- Diarrhea and constipation

15.4 Mechanisms of Action

- It is unknown by what mechanism apples may affect lung function or lower the risk of lung cancer. It has been proposed that the antioxidant flavonoid quercetin may play a major role.[43,178]

- Pectins and pectin-like rhamnogalacturonans have pronounced antimutagenic effects against 1-nitropyrene induced mutagenicity in vitro.[123] *In vitro*, pectin polysaccharides most likely interact directly with cells (*Salmonella typhimurium*) to sterically protect them from mutagenic attack.

- Apple pectin decreases incidence and number of dimethylhydrazine- and azoxymethane-induced colon tumors in rats.[245,325,326] It is thought that pectin lowers β-glucuronidase activity, a key enzymatic step in carcinogen activation and tumor initiation in the colon.

- In the intestine, apple pectin is a bulk forming agent similar to psyllium and prevents diarrhea and constipation by a similar mechanism.

• Pectin may modify intestinal bacterial enzyme activity in favor of a reduction of toxic breakdown products in the gut.[200] This may contribute to a chemoprotective effect in colon carcinogenesis.

15.5 Research

15.5.1 Apple Pectin in Lung Function and Lung Cancer

Researchers[178] found a statistically significant inverse relationship between lung cancer risk and food sources high in the isoflavone quercetin (onions and apples) after controlling for smoking and intakes of saturated fat and β-carotene in a population-based, case-controlled study conducted in Hawaii (Table 15.1).

A long-term cross-sectional analysis of a cohort of 2512 Welshmen aged 45-59 living in Caerphilly, Wales between 1979 and 1983 found that lung function was linearly associated with dietary apple intake (Table 15.2).[43]

This study additionally found that the age-related decline in lung function over five years in these men was offset by consuming five or more apples per week during the study period.[43]

	Q1 (lowest)	Q2	Q3	Q4 (highest)	Two-sided P for trend
Apple	1.0	0.9 (0.6-1.4)	1.0 (0.6-1.6)	0.6 (0.4-1.0)	0.03
Onion	1.0	1.4 (0.9-2.3)	0.9 (0.5-1.4)	0.5 (0.3-0.9)	0.001
Red wine (tertiles)	1.0	0.8 (0.4-1.8)	0.7 (0.4-1.2)	-	0.20
Soy products	1.0	1.6 (1.0-2.7)	1.2 (0.7-2.2)	1.0 (0.5-1.8)	0.28

Table 15.1
Odds ratio for lung cancer in the highest vs. the lowest quartiles for apple intake in a Hawaiian population. An odds ratio of 1.0 indicates no difference (Q1). Parentheses indicate 95% CI. Other foods high in isoflavones are shown for comparison. Of these, only apples and onions are high in quercetin. Adapted from Le Marchand et al.[178]

15.6 Overview

These clinical results coupled with the results of earlier trials strongly suggest that **apple pectin:**

- Protects against cancer, primarily lung cancer
- Improves lung function

15.6.1 Contraindications

- None known

15.6.2 Side Effects

- No adverse reactions are known to occur with consumption of apple fruit or isolated pectin. However, apple seeds contain potentially toxic levels of hydrogen cyanide that, if used incorrectly, can be dangerous.

Difference in lung function (95% CI)				
Frequency of apple consumption	N	Adjusted for age and height	Adjusted for body mass index, and smoking	Adjusted for social class, work exercise, and leisure exercise	Adjusted for total energy intake
None	645	0(baseline)	0 (baseline)	0 (baseline)	0 (baseline)
1	270	97.1(3.2-191.0)	75.7(-15.7-167.1)	49.3(-40.9-139.5)	44.5
2-4	753	159.9(90.2-229.5)	102.9(34.6-171.1)	84.7(17.2-152.1)	88.0
≥5	433	291.8(211.2-372.4)	185.7(104.9-266.5)	146.6(66.5-226.8)	138.1
Test for trend		P<0.001	P<0.001	P<0.001	P<0.001

Table 15.2

Cross-sectional analysis: Differences in forced expiratory volume in one second (FEV1) in mL associated with increases in the frequency of apple intake from baseline. Adapted from Butland et al.[43]

15.6.3 Possible Interactions with Drugs

- None known

15.6.4 Possible Interactions with Herbs and other Dietary Supplements

- Insufficient reliable information available

15.6.5 Possible Interactions with Diseases or Conditions

- None known

15.6.6 Typical Dosage

- **Oral:** 500 mg apple pectin in capsules taken daily or "an apple a day."

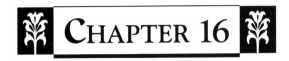

CHAPTER 16

BURDOCK ROOT

Arctium lappa

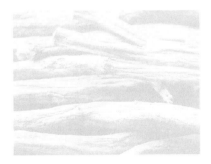

16
~~>>)*(<<~~

BURDOCK ROOT

Arctium lappa

16.1 Description and Medical History

Burdock is a common wild herb native to North America, Europe, and Asia. The plant is typically about 3-5 feet tall with large, ovate leaves. The broad flower heads consist of reddish or violet tubular florets surrounded by numerous hooked bracts that give them a burr-like appearance. The roots are considered the medicinally active part, although the flowers and seeds are sometimes used.

Burdock root has been used in folk medicine to treat colds, catarrh, cancers, and as an aphrodisiac. It also has been used to treat gout and syphilitic disorders. Native Americans made a root poultice to put on boils and abesses.[105] It is commonly consumed as a food in Asia.[141]

Taken orally, burdock is considered a diuretic and "blood purifier," facilitating the removal of toxins from the body via the elimination organs (liver, kidneys, and intestine).[141] It also has antimicrobial and antipyretic (fever reducing) activities. The plant contains arctiopiricin known to be active against Gram-positive bacteria.[141]

Burdock is an ingredient in at least two herbal therapies for cancer. These are Essiac, a commercial remedy of Native American

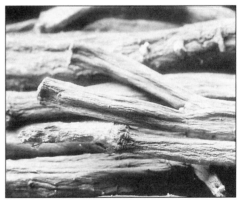

Figure 16.1
Arctium lappa (Burdock Root)

origin[227] discovered by the infamous Canadian nurse, Rene Caisse (1888-1978), and the controversial herbal cancer treatments of Harry Hoxsey (Hoxsey was attacked by the medical establishment as fraudulent in the 1950s but was later vindicated to some extent).[358] Scientists have found a metabolically stable desmutagenic factor in burdock.[89,222] The high molecular weight burdock factor (B-factor) was effective *in vitro* on various types of mutagens in the presence or absence of metabolic activation.[222] There is insufficient clinical evidence available to determine burdock's effectiveness as an anticancer agent *in vivo*.[128]

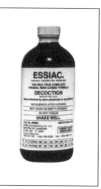

The research literature also suggests that burdock root is gastro- and hepatoprotective, anti-urolithic, and antioxidant.[109,155,189,191]

16.2 Known Medicinal Constituents

- Arctiin and arctigenin and their derivatives
- Chlorogenic and isochlorogenic acids
- Lignans
- Polysaccharides: *inulin, xyloglucans, and acidic xylans*
- Complex mixture of volatile oils: *phenylacetaldehyde, benzaldehyde, 2-alkyl-3-methoxy-pyrazines, and others*
- Essential fatty acids

16.3 Indications for Use

- Clinical Purification[189,191,109,141,155]
- Cancer[89,222,223,340]
- Ailments and complaints of the gastrointestinal tract (empirical data only)
- Inflammatory disorders such as rheumatism, gout, and cystitis[259]
- Skin conditions such as atopic dermatitis, acne, psoriasis, ichthyosis, and eczema (empirical data only)
- Immune system depression (empirical data only)
- Anorexia nervosa (empirical data only)

16.4 Mechanisms of Action

- Arctiin and arctigenin have been shown to be cytotoxic to tumor cells *in vitro* and *in vivo*.[223,340]
- The leaf and flower of burdock are active against Gram-positive and Gram-negative bacteria. The root is primarily active against Gram-negative bacteria.[141]
- Burdock contains inulin that activates the alternate complement pathway (ACP) on which serum bactericidal activity depends. Inulin may help restore this activity as well as increase levels of cyclic-AMP (cAMP) and decrease histamine release.[259]

16.5 Research

16.5.1 Antimutagenic Effect of Burdock Factor

Morita et al[222] isolated a high molecular weight factor from burdock that reduced the mutagenicity in *Salmonella typhimurium* strains TA98 and TA100 of mutagens that are independent of metabolic activation as well as mutagens requiring S9 for activation.

Mutagen	Metabolic activator	Dose (µg/plate)	Number of revertants/plate	
			Without B-factor	With B-factor
4-NO$_2$-1,2-DAB	-	40	1487	584
4-NO$_2$-1,2-DAB	S9	40	909	392
2-NO$_2$-1,4-DAB	-	80	272	49
2-NO2-1,4-DAB	S9	80	614	46
AF-2	-	0.2	349	402
Ethidium bromide	S9	10	909	32
2-aminoanthracene	S9	4	2832	61
Trp-P-1	S9	0.2	1186	53
Trp-P-2	S9	0.2	1046	52

Table 16.1
Desmutagenic effects of burdock root juice (B-factor) on various mutagens.[222]

Table 16.1 summarizes the results of this study. With the exception of 2-(2-furyl)-3-(nitrofuryl)acrylamide (AF-2), the burdock factor exhibited significant desmutagenic effects on all mutagens tested.

The desmutagenic factor also was shown to be heat resistant and extremely stable in the presence of proteolytic enzymes. Interestingly, the factor was active in the presence of Mg^{2+} and Ca^{2+} ions but lost its desmutagenic activity when treated with manganese ions.

Chromatography and spectrophotometry revealed that the burdock factor is a high molecular weight (>300 kD) polyanionic substance with an absorption wavelength of 280-300 nm. Its highly anionic character, coupled with the fact that the B-factor reduces mutagenicity in a dose dependent manner, suggest that it inactivates mutagens by a process of adsorption.

16.5.2 Burdock Root Free Radical Scavenging Activity

Superoxide and hydroxyl radical scavenging activity assays performed by Lin et al,[189] indicate that a freeze-dried aqueous extract of burdock root possesses superoxide radical scavenging activity similar to superoxide dismutase (burdock extract IC_{50}=2.06 mg/mL) and hydroxyl radical scavenging activity similar to ascorbic acid (burdock extract IC_{50}=11.8 mg/mL). In addition, *the extract was shown to significantly reduce carrageenan-induced paw edema in rats similar to indomethacin, a standard anti-inflammatory agent* (Table 16.2). The extract also reduced CCl_4-induced hepatotoxicity in a dose dependant manner, as measured by serum glutamine-oxaloacetic transaminase (GOT) and glutamic-pyruvic transaminase (GPT) levels (Table 16.3). Additionally, burdock root extract reduced the degree of centrilobular necrosis and cellular architecture loss in the liver.

Group	Extract Dose (mg/kg, s.c.)	Edema (%) (mean±SE)	Inhibition rate (%)
Control (saline)	-	47.47±1.77	-
Burdock (low)	100	36.87±0.58*	22.33
Burdock (medium)	300	36.08±1.18*	23.99
Burdock (high)	1000	35.60±1.84*	25.01
Indomethacin	10	31.23±0.77*	34.21

* (P<0.01)

Table 16.2
Effect of burdock extracts and indomethacin on carrageenan-induced paw edema in rats.[189]

Group	Extract Dose (mg/kg)	GOT (IU/L)	GPT (IU/L)
Control (saline)	-	85.32±2.00	22.20±0.26
CCl$_4$	-	226.82±24.16[a]	56.30±2.73[a]
CCl$_4$/Burdock (low)	100	149.93±14.91[b]	37.55±2.88[c]
CCl$_4$/Burdock (medium)	300	95.03±5.64[c]	20.93±1.24[c]
CCl$_4$/Burdock (high)	1000	79.25±5.43[c]	14.55±0.59[c]
Silymarin	25	113.62±6.43[c]	34.82±1.17[c]

[a] (P<0.01), significantly different from normal control   [b] (P<0.05), significantly different from CCl4-treated group
[c] (P<0.01), significantly different from CCl4-treated group

Table 16.3
Hepatoprotective effects of burdock on the CCl4-induced GOT and GPT level increase.[189]

Assay	Blank	Control	CCl4	CCl4 + burdock
SGOT (IU/L)	91.83±10.65	97.25±13.11	5405.0±1134.29[a]	383.13±60.77[1]
SGPT (IU/L)	70.70±2.80	58.90±5.90	6632.33±740.34[a]	564.14±50.80[1]
Glutathione (mmol/gm liver)	14.16±0.21	12.85±0.43	6.04±0.33[a]	7.34±0.31[3]
Malondialdehyde (mg/g protein)	0.75±0.08	1.11±0.26	1.77±0.16[c]	1.13±0.15[2]
Cytochrome P450 (nmol/mg protein)	0.62±0.03	0.52±0.01	0.27±0.03[a]	0.50±0.02[1]
Cytochrome b5 (nmol/mg protein)	0.27±0.01	0.29±0.01	0.21±0.01[b]	0.24±0.01[3]
NADPH-cytochrome C reductase (nmol cyt. C reduced/mg protein/min)	21.28±0.63	21.79±0.08	14.37±1.34[b]	20.84±2.48[3]

a (P<0.001), significantly different from control   1 (P<0.001), significantly different from CCl4 group
b (P<0.01), significantly different from control   2 (P<0.01), significantly different from CCl4 group
c (P<0.05), significantly different from control   3 (P<0.05), significantly different from CCl4 group

Table 16.4
Burdock extract (300 mg/kg, oral) protected against acute
liver damage induced by CCl4 (32 mL/kg, i.p.) poisoning in mice.[191]

Lin et al[191] also showed that burdock was chemoprotective against CCl_4- and acetominophen-induced liver damage. Burdock reversed the depletion of glutathione induced by these chemicals and normalized the levels of cytochrome P-450, cytochrome b5, and NADPH-cytochrome C reductase. Tables 16.4 and 16.5 summarize these results.

Liver injury due to CCl_4 is attributed to the production of free radicals and membrane lipid peroxidation. The results of these studies suggest that burdock functions as an effective chemoprotector by increasing endogenous levels of antioxidant molecules such as glutathione and by successfully scavenging superoxide and hydroxyl radicals.

Assay	Blank	Control	Acetominophen	Acetominophen + burdock
SGOT (IU/L)	85.17±14.67	101.25±11.16	730.33±155.25[a]	178.30±21.34[1]
SGPT (IU/L)	75.13±15.10	76.60±5.90	2665.80±794.76[a]	111.29±12.72[1]
Glutathione (mmol/gm liver)	19.5±0.67	19.40±0.92	8.43±0.45[a]	11.01±0.67[1]
Malondialdehyde (mg/g protein)	0.45±0.03	0.44±0.03	0.81±0.06[b]	0.44±0.01[2]
Cytochrome P450 (nmol/mg protein)	0.68±0.01	0.62±0.04	0.29±0.01[b]	0.44±0.01[2]
Cytochrome b5 (nmol/mg protein)	0.26±0.01	0.31±0.06	0.17±0.01[b]	0.25±0.01[2]
NADPH-cytochrome C reductase (nmol cyt. C reduced/mg protein/min)	19.97±0.86	18.92±0.67	14.80±2.20	21.36±0.95[1]

[a]($P<0.05$), significantly different from control   [1]($P<0.05$), significantly different from acetominophen group

[b]($P<0.001$), significantly different from control   [2]($P<0.001$), significantly different from acetominophen group

Table 16.5
*Burdock extract (300 mg/kg, oral) protected against acute liver
damage induced by acetominophen (600 mg/kg, i.p.) poisoning in mice.*[191]

16.6 Overview

These clinical results coupled with the results of other trials strongly suggest that **burdock:**

- Is antimutagenic against both metabolism-dependent and independent mutagens
- Acts as an antioxidant in protecting cellular tissues against peroxidation
- Is hepatoprotective

16.6.1 Contraindications

- Burdock is contraindicated with allergic sensitivity to the Asteraceae/Compositae family: *ragweed, chrysanthemum, marigold, daisy, and others.*[141]
- Topically, skin sensitivity is possible.[88,141,272]

16.6.2 Side Effects

- Dietary burdock aggravated the diabetic condition in a study of streptozotocin diabetic mice.[318] However, this contradicts burdock's hypoglycemic activity cited in other studies.
- Anticholinergic poisonings have been associated with commercial burdock root tea.[269] This was found to be a result of contamination with atropine.
- Burdock has antiplatelet activity and may increase the risk of bleeding in some people.[137]

16.6.3 Possible Interactions with Drugs

- Burdock in large quantities may have a hypoglycemic effect interfering with hypoglycemic drugs.[141]
- Concomitant use with insulin may require insulin dose adjustment due to hypoglycemic effect.[141]
- Use of burdock may interfere with antiplatelet/anticoagulant drugs and may increase the risk of bleeding in some people.[137]

16.6.4 Possible Interactions with Herbs and other Dietary Supplements

• There is insufficient reliable information on burdock's interaction with other herbs and dietary supplements.[141]

16.6.5 Typical Dosage

• **Oral:** 2-6 grams of the dried root three times daily. Tea: steep 1-2 grams of the dried root in 150 mL boiling water for 5-10 minutes; one cup, strained, three times daily. Liquid extract: (1:1 in 25% alcohol) 2-8 mL three times daily. Tincture: (1:10 in 45% alcohol) 8-12 mL three times daily (141). When used as part of a synergistic detoxification formula: 100 to 250 mg, 3 times per day.

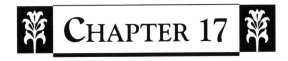

CHAPTER 17

RED CLOVER

Trifolium pratense

17

⇥⇥⟫⟨⟨⟨

RED CLOVER

Trifolium pratense

17.1 Description and Medical History

Red clover is a wild legume indigenous to Europe, central Asia, and north Africa that has become naturalized in North America and many other parts of the world.[30]

The plant is a perennial herb 15-40 cm tall with a bushy rhizome and a basal leaf rosette.[88] The flowers, globular and ovate, range in color from light carmine to red and form on the tips of the stems. Occasionally, the flowers may be yellowish or white.[88] The leaves of red clover are elliptical or ovate and have a characteristic "arrow-shaped" white spot on the upper surface. The leaves are trifoliate which is the basis for the Latin name of the plant.

Red clover contains phytoestrogens, naturally occurring compounds that resemble hormones and appear to mimic them *in vivo*[235,385,386] Indeed, red clover can cause fertility "disturbances" in cattle grazed on it.[146,243,244] The medicinal parts of the plant are the fresh and dried flower buds.

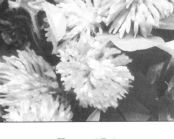

Figure 17.1
Trifolium pratense (Red Clover)

17.2 Known Medicinal Constituents

- Isoflavones: *biochanin A, formononetin and derivatives genistein and daidzein*
- Coumarins[88,141]
- Volatile oils and tannins[88,141]

17.3 Indications for Use

- Clinical Purification[168,214]
- Atherosclerosis and arterial hypertension[74,75,87,235]
- Certain hormone-related and other cancers[45,71,97,122,133]
- Photo-induced skin cancer[367,371]
- Hyperlipidemia and hypercholesterolemia[108,293]
- Lipid peroxidation[104,274,334]
- Some menopausal symptomology[141,170,235]
- Externally: *Psoriasis, eczema, and certain other skin conditions* (effectiveness unverified by clinical research studies)[88,141]
- Respiratory ailments: *whooping cough, cough, asthma, and bronchitis* (folk medicine, not clinically verified)[141]

17.4 Mechanisms of Action

- The phytoestrogenic isoflavones contained in red clover are thought to weakly mimic the actions of sex hormones in the body, primarily estrogen and estradiol.[235,385,386] This is the likely mechanism for the positive action of phytoestrogens observed in post-menopausal women.[71,133,235,385] However, in premenopausal women the isoflavones may act as both hormone agonists and antagonists because they compete with estrogen and estradiol for cellular estrogen receptors.[386] *Isoflavones may protect against toxic environmental estrogens, such as pesticides, by competitively binding cellular estrogen receptors.*[168,214] Lignans and isoflavonoids have been shown to stimulate the synthesis of sex hormone binding globulin in the liver, suggesting another means by which isoflavones may regulate sex hormone activity.[4,5]

- Some research evidence suggests that biochanin A mediates red clover's cardioprotective action by inhibiting the abnormal growth of cardiac fibroblasts and aortic smooth muscle cells

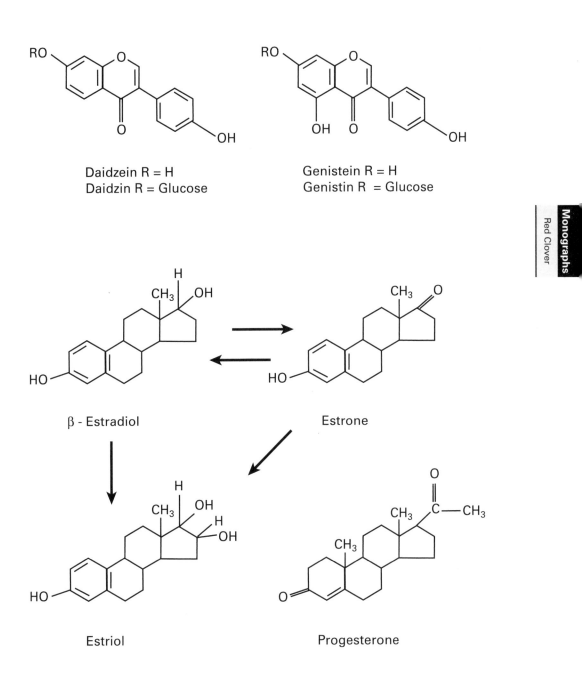

Daidzein R = H
Daidzin R = Glucose

Genistein R = H
Genistin R = Glucose

β - Estradiol

Estrone

Estriol

Progesterone

Figure 17.2
Structural similarities between estrogen/estradiol, biochanin A/formononetin and genistein/daidzein.

evident in cardiovascular disease[74,75] Isoflavones also have been shown to relax rabbit coronary arteries *in vitro* by a calcium dependent mechanism.[87]

• Several purified isoflavones have shown chemoprotective effects in cancer studies.[48,45,371] The isoflavones may exert their putative anticancer action via estrogenic and nonestrogenic pathways.[133,268,351,359,378] Phytoestrogens have antimutagenic activity in vitro[92,93,367] and isoflavones such as genistein have been shown to inhibit tyrosine protein kinases involved in receptor-mediated cell growth stimulation and oncogene activation.[8]

• *In vitro*, purified isoflavones significantly increase expression of metallothionein (an antioxidant protein) in cultured human colon cells.[147] Because they have a phenolic structure, isoflavones may act as antioxidants, either by preventing metabolism of procarcinogens to carcinogens or by eliminating free radicals.[232,366]

• Red clover contains many of the same lignans and isoflavones as soybean and other legumes. Both biochanin A and formononetin can be converted to genistein and daidzein, respectively, by *Eubacterium limosum*, an anaerobic bacterium found in the human intestinal tract.[10,134] The latter isoflavones are main active constituents of soybeans. Although less research has been done on red clover, its isoflavones may provide some of the same chemoprotective and antioxidant actions as clinical studies have shown with soy isoflavones.[10,170,315]

• There is little evidence to support red clover's use in asthma and respiratory disease. However, dietary phytoestrogens were shown to be anti-inflammatory in a guinea pig model of asthma.[267]

17.5 Research

Epidemiological investigations and clinical studies point to phytoestrogen-containing foods as chemoprotective agents. Table 17.1 presents a summary of this research, as collected by Adlercreutz et al.[8]

Researchers such as Adlercreutz et al[8,9] postulate that the Western diet, compared with vegetarian or semivegetarian diets in developing countries and Asia, may alter hormone production, metabolism, and/or action at the cellular level. Their studies and others illustrate the view that the Western diet is one of the main factors causing so-called "Western diseases," such as

Type of cancer	Compound or food	Test subjects	Effect or results
Breast	Genistein	MCF-7 cells	Competition with estradiol[203]
Breast	Diet and phytoestrogen excretion	Women	Low urinary excretion in women at higher risk[2]
Breast	Diet and phytoestrogen excretion	Women	Low urinary excretion in women at higher risk[3]
Breast	Diet and phytoestrogen excretion	Finnish, American, and Japanese women	Correlation with plasma sex hormone binding globulin[4]
(VAL 12) Ha-ras-transformed cells	Genistein	NIH 3T3 cells	Inhibition of proliferation[246]
Breast	Diet and phytoestrogen excretion	Women	Lowest urinary excretion in breast cancer patients[5]
Prostate	Soy products	Men of Japanese ancestry	Less risk[291]
Mitogen-induced proliferation	Daidzein	Human lymphocytes	Inhibition of proliferation[125]
Breast	Daidzein	ZR-75-1 cells	Inhibition[126]
Erythroleukemia	Genistein	Mouse MEL cells	Induction of Differentiation[363]
Breast	Soybean chips, heated and non-heated	Rat	Inhibition of tumor growth[25]
Melanoma	Genistein	Five cell lines	Differentiation[161]
Myeloid leukemia	Genistein	Human K562 cells	Differentiation[130]
Breast	Flaxseed	Rat	Protective[288,333]
Colon	Flaxseed	Rat	Protective[289,333]
Leukemia	Genistein	Human HL-60, K-562 cells	Differentiation[60]

Table 17.1 (continued on next page)
Studies related to possible anticancer effects of isoflavonoids and lignans found in phytoestrogen-containing foods.[8]

Type of cancer	Compound or food	Test subjects	Effect or results
Breast	Soy food	Women in Singapore	High intake associated with low risk[179]
Myeloid leukemia	Genistein	ML-1, HL-60 cells	Differentiation[198]
Myeloid leukemia	Genistein	MO7E cells	Inhibition of proliferation[169]
Prostatic dysplasia	Soy food	Male mice	Inhibition[197]
Breast	Genistein, Biochanin A	MCF-7 and other human cells	Inhibition of proliferation[253]
Embryonal carcinoma	Genistein	Mouse F9 cells	Differentiation[165]
Breast	Heated soybean protein isolate	Rat	Inhibition of tumor progression[118]
Mitogen-induced proliferation	Plant lignans	Human lymphocytes	Inhibition of proliferation[127]
Normal cells	Biochanin A	Embryonic hamster cells	Decreased metabolism of benzo[a]pyrene[50]
Breast	Enterolactone	MCF-7 cells	Inhibition of proliferation in the presence of estradiol[228]
Prostatitis	Soy food	Rat	Preventive effect[295]
Leukemia	Genistein	MOLT-4, HL-60 human cells	Inhibits cell cycle progression and growth[336]
Breast cancer	Flaxseed	Rat	Inhibits the promotional phase[290]
Solid pediatric tumors	Genistein	Neuroblastoma, sarcoma cells	Inhibition of proliferation[286]
Liver	Enterolactone	HepG2 cells	Stimulation of sex hormone binding globulin synthesis[6]
Non-P-glycoprotein-mediated multidrug resistant cells	Genistein	K562/TPA	Reversal of Resistance[322]

Table 17.1 (continued on next page)

Studies related to possible anticancer effects of isoflavonoids and lignans found in phytoestrogen-containing foods.[8]

Type of cancer	Compound or food	Test subjects	Effect or results
Leukemia and TPA-stimulated PNM cells	Genistein	HL-60 and TPA-stimulated PMN cells	Inhibition of hydrogen peroxide formation[366]
Placental microsomes	Lignans	Human	Inhibition of aromatase[7]
Endothelial cells	Genistein	Many different endothelial cells	Inhibition of angiogenesis[91]
Myeloid leukemia	Daidzein	HL-60 cells	Differentiation[143]
Non-P-glycoprotein-mediated multidrug resistant cells	Genistein	Many different cell types	Modulation of decreased drug accumulation[353]
Gastric	Genistein	HGC-27 cells	Growth inhibition[206]
Monoblastic leukemia	Genistein	U937 cells	Differentiation[199]
Liver	Genistein	HepG2 cells	Inhibition of proliferation[229]
Prostate	Genistein	LNCaP, DU-145 cells	Inhibition of proliferation[254]
Colon	Soy	Japanese men and women	Reduced risk[364]
Gastric, esophagus, colon	Genistein, biochanin A	Many types of cells	Inhibition of proliferation; apoptosis[376]
Preadipocytes	Biochanin A	Human	Inhibition of aromatase[45]
TPA-mediated skin tumor	Genistein	Mouse	Inhibition[366]
Monocytic leukemia	Genistein	Mouse cell line	Cytotoxicity[148]
Lymphoma	Genistein	Rat Nb2 lymphoma cells	Growth inhibition[38]

Table 17.1 (continued from previous page)
Studies related to possible anticancer effects of isoflavonoids and lignans found in phytoestrogen-containing foods.[8]

Results				
Population/ dietary group	Number of subjects	Total urinary lignans (µmol/day)	Total urinary isoflavonoids (nmol/day)	Total urinary diphenols (µmol/day)
Premenopausal Finnish Women				
Omnivores	12	2.89 (2.53-3.30)	391 (325-470)	3.40 (3.03-3.83)
Vegetarians	11	4.16 (3.34-5.18)	665 (469-944)	5.59 (4.55-6.86)
Breast Cancer	10	2.34 (1.88-2.90)	279 (241-324)	2.70 (2.19-3.32)
Postmenopausal Finnish Women				
Omnivores	10	1.99 (1.64-2.41)	95.3 (78.0-116)	2.14 (1.79-2.56)
Vegetarians	10	8.09 (5.19-12.6)	323 (225-462)	9.33 (6.05-14.4)
Breast Cancer	10	2.08 (1.54-2.82)	94.2 (67.5-132)	2.27 (1.68-3.08)
Premenopausal American Women				
Omnivores	10	2.22 (1.92-2.57)	515 (443-600)	2.83 (2.49-3.22)
Vegetarians	10	6.78 (4.92-9.33)	1862 (1585-2188)	9.35 (7.18-12.2)
Macrobiotics	13	28.8 (23.0-36.1)	6855 (5508-8531)	38.4 (31.3-47.0)
Prostmenopausal American Women				
Omnivores	11	2.07 (1.69-2.54)	178 (142-223)	2.46 (2.05-2.95)
Vegetarians	12	1.9 (1.15-3.13)	1282 (885-1858)	3.47 (2.34-5.14)
Macrobiotics	7	24.5 (16.3-37.0)	5470 (3412-8770)	34.0 (24.3-47.6)

Table 17.2
Urinary total lignan, isoflavonoid, and diphenol excretion in various populations and dietary groups. Data summarized from Adlercreutz et al[8]

the major hormone-dependent cancers, colon cancer, and coronary heart disease. These researchers suggest that the high levels of isoflavones found in non-Western diets decrease the risk of disease. Table 17.2 contains epidemiological data supporting this hypothesis. Vegetarians and people consuming a macrobiotic diet show greater urinary isoflavone and lignan excretion than omnivores. Furthermore, as a trend, breast cancer survivors show the lowest urinary excretion of all.[8]

17.5.1 Antioxidant Activity of Phytoestrogens

High consumption of foods rich in phytoestrogens has been linked epidemiologically to reduced incidence of cancers at many sites. One hypothesis is that *the anticarcinogenic activity of phytoestrogens involves induction of detoxifying Phase II enzymes.*

Biochanin A and genistein both increase NADPH:quinone reductase (QR) activity and mRNA expression in cultured colon cancer cells (360; Colo205 cells).

Researchers[274] measured the total antioxidant activity of solutions of several phytoestrogens spectrophotometrically relative to standard solutions of Trolox, a powerful antioxidant. The ability of the phytoestrogens to reduce 2,2'-azinobis(3)-ethylbenzothiazoline-6-sulphonic acid

Results	
Isoflavone	**TEAC (Mm)**
Genistin	1.24±0.02
Genistein	2.90±0.10
Biochanin A	1.16±0.02
Daidzein	1.25±0.02
Formononetin	0.11±0.02
Daidzin	1.15±0.01
Ononin	0.05±0.04

Table 17.3
Total antioxidant activity of several isoflavones using the ABTS$^{+\bullet}$ total antioxidant spectrophotometric assay. Trolox Equivalent Antioxidant Capacity (TEAC) is the millimolar concentration of a Trolox solution having an antioxidant capacity equivalent to a 1.0 mM solution of the substance under investigation. Thus, a TEAC value > 1 indicates strong antioxidant activity.[274]

radical (ABTS$^{+\bullet}$) relative to Trolox is shown in Table 17.3. Genistein had an antioxidant activity in this assay nearly three times that of Trolox or Vitamin C.

In the same study, these phytoestrogens also protected LDL cholesterol from oxidation by copper ions.

Human cytochrome P450 3A4 (CYP 3A4) is a detoxification enzyme found in high amounts in liver and epithelial tissue of the small intestine. It is a major contributor to the presystemic metabolism of orally administered drugs and has wide substrate specificity in the gut. Grapefruit juice is one known inhibitor of this enzyme, accounting for the increased oral availability of drugs consumed with grapefruit juice.[95,120,193] A commercially available extract of red clover herb and flower buds (55% ethanol) was shown to strongly inhibit CYP 3A4 metabolism of the assay test substrate 7-benzyloxyresorufin.[40] Red clover extract inhibited the enzyme dose-dependently and had an IC_{50}=1.05% of full strength (R^2=0.90).

This result suggests that red clover may facilitate the uptake of drugs and herbal medicines by inhibiting intestinal CYP 3A4 that would normally metabolize them. In addition, inhibition of liver CYP 3A4 may prolong the effects of other active molecules in the body.[95]

17.5.2 Cardioprotective Action of Phytoestrogens

Smooth muscle cells (SMCs) contribute to the structural changes that occur in blood vessel walls[75] in vasoocclusive cardiovascular diseases such as atherosclerosis. SMCs migrate from the media to the intima of the blood vessels, proliferate, and deposit extracellular matrix (ECM) molecules such as collagen, which causes thickening and occlusion of the blood vessels.

The isoflavones biochanin A, genistein, equol, daidzein, and formononetin inhibit the *in vitro* DNA synthesis, proliferation, collagen synthesis, total protein synthesis, and migration of SMCs.[75] These behaviors are essential to neointima formation in hypertension, atherosclerosis, and coronary artery disease, *suggesting that natural dietary phytoestrogens offer significant protection from these diseases.* Indeed, the human plasma levels of phytoestrogens from the diet have been measured at above 4 μmol/L,[226] well within the effective concentration range used *in vitro*.

The researchers also found that the primary action of the isoflavones on SMCs is not, in fact, estrogen receptor-mediated. Daidzein, biochanin A, and genistein inhibit MAP kinase activity in these cells. This enzyme is a key element in the mitogenic biochemical pathway of SMCs.

17.6 Overview

These clinical results coupled with the results of earlier trials strongly suggest that **red clover:**

- Is a chemoprotecive agent
- Induces phase II liver detoxification enzymes
- Supports cardiovascular health
- Functions as an antioxidant

17.6.1 Contraindications

- Avoid using red clover in large amounts in blood coagulation disorders.[121,141]
- Avoid using red clover in large amounts in fertility or sex hormone-related conditions.[141]

Note: this contraindication is controversial and warrants further research.

17.6.2 Side Effects

- Theoretically, the phytoestrogens can stimulate estrogen-like activity. Large quantitiesof red clover are known to induce sterility in livestock,[141,146] but this has not been documented in humans.

17.6.3 Possible Interactions with Drugs

- Concomitant use of large amounts of red clover with antiplatelet/anticoagulant drugs may increase the risk of bleeding in some people due to red clover's high coumarin content.[141]
- In theory, large amounts of red clover may interfere with hormone replacement therapy or oral contraceptives via competition of phytoestrogens for sex hormone receptors.[141]

17.6.4 Possible Interactions with Herbs and other Dietary Supplements

- Concomitant use of coumarin-containing herbs may increase the risk of bleeding in some people due to the anticoagulant effect of coumarins.
- Red clover may be additive or possibly antagonistic with other herbs with estrogenic activity.

17.6.5 Possible Interactions with Diseases or Conditions

• Coagulation disorders: Use red clover with caution and avoid large amounts because coumarin content may increase the risk of bleeding.

• Estrogen-sensitive conditions: Because red clover contains phytoestrogens thought to have estrogenic properties, these could interact with diseases or conditions sensitive to such ingredients.

17.6.6 Typical Dosage

• **Oral:** Typically 4 grams of the flower tops three times daily or one cup of the tea (4 grams in 150 mL boiling water for 10-15 minutes) three times daily. Liquid extract (1:1 in 25% ethanol): 1.5-3 mL three times daily. Tincture (1:10 in 45% ethanol): 1-2 mL three times daily. When used as part of a synergistic detoxification formula: 100 to 300 mg of dried herb, 3 times per day.

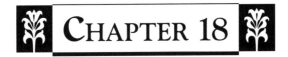

CHAPTER 18

PSYLLIUM

Plantago ovata

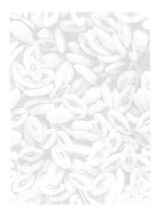

18
⇒⟫✳⟪⇐

Psyllium

Plantago ovata

18.1 Description and Medical History

Blonde psyllium husk is a rich source of concentrated soluble fiber shown to significantly reduce cholesterol in humans and animals.[19,21,167] In fact, as revealed in Table 18.1, numerous studies confirm that psyllium has the strongest activity in reducing serum and liver lipid levels when compared to other popular fiber sources.

Recommendations for dietary fiber intake for adults are 20-35 g/day or 10-13 g/1,000 kcal. However, common serving sizes of grain, fruit, and vegetables contain only 1-3 grams of dietary fiber.[304] Psyllium can serve as a supplemental fiber source to maintain recommended fiber intake.

Psyllium is an annual plant that grows naturally in India, Afghanistan, Iran, Israel, northern Africa, Spain, and the Canary Islands.[88] It is cultivated in India and neighboring countries, Arizona, and southern Brazil.

As a dietary supplement, psyllium refers to the ripe seeds or ground seed epidermis. **Psyllium's contribution to detoxification is largely via improved intestinal function and reduction of liver and serum total and LDL cholesterol.**

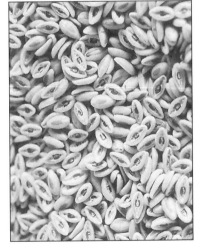

Figure 18.1
Plantago ovato (Psyllium seeds)

18.2 Known Medicinal Constituents (Psyllium seed husk)

- Mucilagenous polysaccharides: highly branched, acidic arabinoxylans

18.3 Indications for Use

- Clinical Purification
- Constipation
- Diarrhea
- Hypercholesterolemia
- Hyperglycemia
- Ulcerative colitis in remission

Fiber type	Number of studies	Serum cholesterol (% change)	Liver cholesterol (% change)	Average cholesterol (% change)	Serum triglyceride (mg/dL)
Psyllium	7	-32±6	-52±5	-42	169±15
Oat gum	11	-22±3	-45±7	-34	169±11
Guar gum	3	-23	-43	-33	NA
Pectin	20	-17±4	-35±6	-26	193±12
Oat bran	8	-12±2	-28±6	-20	162±14
Soy fiber	6	-11±2	-17±3	-14	168±15
Corn bran	2	-6	-11	-9	105
Cellulose	26	0	0	0	187±13
Wheat bran	5	-1±11	+6±1	+2	116±12

Adapted from Anderson et al.[19] Values expressed as mean±SEM. Cholesterol values represent the percentage change from cellulose (control) values in the same experiment. Average cholesterol change is the average of serum and liver cholesterol changes. Triglyceride values are averages from the number of studies indicated.

Table 18.1
Response of serum and liver cholesterol and serum triglyceride values to intake of various fibers in a rat model.[19]

18.4 Mechanisms of Action

Psyllium seed husk can absorb 8 to 14 times its weight in water. The fibrous quality makes psyllium a bulk-forming laxative in cases of constipation, stimulating peristalsis and shortening intestinal transit time. Ironically, its absorptive quality also can stop diarrhea by taking up extra liquid in the intestine and prolonging intestinal transit time. Psyllium tends to swell in the intestine creating a feeling of fullness that can reduce appetite.[141] Intestinal flora can ferment psyllium and other soluble fibers into short-chain fatty acids, primarily butyrate, which are known to support maintenance of intestinal epithelial cell populations, facilitate epithelium repair, and suppress epithelial nuclear factor kappa B-DNA binding activity,[86,149] thus promoting intestinal health and repair. Butyrate has antineoplastic properties against colorectal cancer and is the preferred substrate for the oxidative reactions of colonocytes.[241]

The preponderance of research evidence suggests that psyllium's cholesterol-lowering activity is due to increased bile acid excretion and concomitant up-regulation of bile acid production from hepatic cholesterol.[41,84,204,337] This mechanism is likely responsible for the gall-stone preventive action of psyllium as well.[337]

Soluble fiber also may act by altering the absorption of cholesterol and fat in the intestine.[98] In addition, the short-chain fatty acids from fermentation of psyllium fiber by gut microflora may inhibit hepatic cholesterol synthesis.[20,53] These proposed mechanisms are not mutually exclusive and may work additively to lower cholesterol.

It has been shown that psyllium must be consumed with a meal in order to show cholesterol-reducing activity.[372] Psyllium taken alone between meals does not appear to significantly reduce serum total, LDL, or HDL cholesterol.

Psyllium is proposed to reduce blood sugar by inhibiting absorption of starch and sugar in the gut.[54,270]

18.5 Research

18.5.1 Psyllium and Gastrointestinal Function

Psyllium seeds may be just as effective as mesalamine for maintaining remission of ulcerative colitis. 105 patients with ulcerative colitis in remission were treated with either 10 grams of psyllium, 500 milligrams of mesalamine, or both. At 12 months the remission failure rates were 40%, 35%, and 30%, respectively; the difference was statistically significant.[86] In addition, fecal butyrate levels were significantly higher after psyllium treatment, suggesting that short-chain fatty acids derived from soluble fiber fermentation play an important role in gastrointestinal health.

18.5.2 Psyllium and Cholesterol

Anderson et al[21] performed a meta-analysis of eight controlled trials on the cholesterol-lowering effects of psyllium husk in mild to moderate hypercholesterolemic humans (Table 18.2). The combined statistical power of the meta-analysis strongly supports the hypothesis that psyllium husk ingestion significantly reduces liver and serum total and LDL cholesterol with little or no change in levels of HDL and triglycerides.[21]

Kritchevsky et al[167] performed a controlled clinical study examining the effect of ground psyllium seed and defatted psyllium husk (as well as pectin and cellulose) on plasma and liver lipids in rats consuming a cholesterol diet. The results are shown in Table 18.3. Defatted psyllium

Results					
	Psyllium group (n=384)		Placebo group (n=272)		Net difference (%)
Serum variable	Baseline	Change	Baseline	Change	(psyllium-placebo)
Total cholesterol (mmol/L)	6.144±0.710	-0.272±0.032[a]	6.230±0.742	-0.034±0.033	-3.87±0.74[c]
LDL cholesterol (mmol/L)	4.189±0.591	-0.298±0.029[a]	4.269±0.611	-0.017±0.030	-6.68±0.96[c]
HDL cholesterol (mmol/L)	1.273±0.310	-0.013±0.009	1.270±0.322	0.000±0.010	-1.04±1.04
Triacylglycerol (mmol/L)	1.491±0.641	0.064±0.029[a]	1.514±0.678	0.008±0.029	3.67±2.78
LDL:HDL ratio	3.49±0.97	-0.21±0.04[a]	3.60±0.95	0.02±0.04	-6.58±1.47[c]
Total: HDL ratio	5.10±1.25	-0.17±0.04[a]	5.20±1.24	0.02±0.05	-3.68±1.22[b]
Apo A-I (g/L)	1.50±0.334	0.0873±0.020	1.48±0.440	0.0397±0.0241	3.18±2.14
Apo B (g/L)	1.31±0.274	0.0172±0.0214	1.33±0.478	0.0058±0.0238	-0.89±2.50
Apo B:apo A-I ratio	0.91±0.26	-0.06±0.01[a]	0.92±0.29	-0.01±0.02	-5.63±2.87[a]

[a] $P<0.05$ [b] $P<0.005$ [c] $P<0.0001$

Table 18.2
Meta-analysis of baseline serum lipid concentrations and post-treatment changes in subjects consuming psyllium or placebo for eight weeks.[21]

husk reduced serum total cholesterol and essentially normalized serum triglycerides, liver weight, and liver lipids of cholesterol fed rats relative to the "normal" levels in rats fed a cholesterol-free diet. HDL was elevated in cholesterol/psyllium husk-fed rats even though total cholesterol was 23% lower than rats fed the cholesterol free diet. Phospholipids also achieved "normal" levels in rats fed psyllium husk.

A review of human studies on soluble fiber by Glore et al[106] lends further support to the clinical data on psyllium and cholesterol (Table 18.4). Most studies reviewed found significant reductions in serum total and LDL cholesterol but no significant changes in HDL and triglyceride levels.[106]

	Basal diet (B)	Basal +0.5% cholesterol (BC)	BC +10% cellulose	BC +10% pectin	BC +10% psyllium seed	BC +10% defatted psyllium husk	ANOVA P<
Weight gain (g)	181±6	188±7	201±10	177±6	182±6	176±5	NS
Liver weight (g)	10.6±0.33	15.9±0.56	15.8±0.80	13.1±0.52	13.1±0.48	11.2±0.28	0.001
Relative liver weight	2.93±0.04	4.32±0.13	4.16±0.15	3.67±0.12	3.62±0.08	3.17±0.07	0.001
Serum (mg/dL)							
Total cholesterol	93±7	112±8	100±3	89±3	87±3	72±3	0.001
HDL cholesterol	46±4.4	45±2.8	47±6.8	46±2.9	53±2.3	51±2.7	NS
%HDL cholesterol	49.7±3.6	41.4±2.2	45.9±3.6	51.2±3.1	61.1±2.1	71.1±3.7	0.001
Triglycerides	46±2	53±2	58±4	65±2	59±2	49±2	0.001
Phospholipids	53±6	73±6	79±6	77±5	81±5	66±5	0.05
Liver (g/100g)							
Total cholesterol	0.71±0.04	4.32±0.18	3.91±0.28	2.55±0.27	1.53±0.12	0.87±0.07	0.001
% ester	64.6±2.54	92.9±0.53	89.2±0.76	90.8±0.69	86.1±1.45	72.4±3.17	0.001
Triglycerides	2.16±0.35	7.15±0.71	6.32±0.46	4.16±0.55	3.45±0.39	2.04±0.25	0.001
Phospholipids	2.89±0.16	2.24±0.10	2.31±0.13	2.55±0.09	2.25±0.06	2.87±0.14	0.001

Monographs
Psyllium

Table 18.3
The influence of psyllium preparations on plasma and liver lipids of cholesterol-fed rats.[167]

Numerous studies have looked at the cholesterol-lowering effects of psyllium in hypercholesterolemic humans on low-fat diets. However, other studies have shown significant reductions in cholesterol in normolipidemic humans and animals on both low and high fat diets.[98,99,167] Furthermore, it has been shown that in human subjects there is no significant difference in the LDL cholesterol response between subjects receiving psyllium on either a high or low fat diet, suggesting the hypocholesterolemic effect is independent of dietary fat content.[307]

Used in conjunction with a low-fat diet, psyllium has been shown to reduce serum total and LDL cholesterol to levels below baseline values for diet alone.[18] It has been estimated that serum cholesterol reductions of 15-19% as observed in some psyllium studies may decrease the risk for coronary heart disease by greater than 30%.[18]

Results			
Reduced serum total cholesterol	Reduced serum LDL	No significant change in serum HDL	No significant change in serum triglycerides
68 of 77 studies analyzed (88%)	41 of 49 studies analyzed (84%)	43 of 57 studies analyzed (75%)	50 of 58 studies analyzed (86%)

Table 18.4
Review of human studies on the effects of soluble fiber on cholesterol.[106]

18.6 Overview

These clinical results coupled with the results of earlier trials strongly suggest that **psyllium:**

- Reduces serum and liver total and LDL cholesterol
- Supports cardiovascular health

18.6.1 Contraindications

- Swallowing difficulties

- Psyllium hypersensitivity
- GI conditions (fecal impaction, atony, GI tract narrowing or obstruction, or spastic bowel)

Note: these conditions may benefit from a synergistic gastrointestinal fiber combination that includes psyllium in combination with foods and herbs that address these conditions.

18.6.2 Side Effects

- In clinical studies, reports of adverse reactions to psyllium are infrequent and do not differ significantly between psyllium and placebo groups.[21] Symptoms involving the digestive system (e.g., flatulence, abdominal pain, diarrhea, constipation, dyspepsia, or nausea) and symptoms of the upper respiratory tract (e.g., rhinitis, infection, pharyngitis, cough increase, or sinusitis) are the most common side effects reported (2-3% of subjects).

- Psyllium can cause allergic reactions in sensitive individuals and is responsible for at least one case of anaphylaxis.[347] However, reports of serious adverse events due to psyllium ingestion are very low in clinical studies.[21]

- Taking psyllium with insufficient water can cause choking.[141]

18.6.3 Possible Interactions with Drugs

- Psyllium may delay intestinal absorption of other drugs taken simultaneously.[88]
- Insulin dosage adjustment (decrease) may be necessary when diabetics use psyllium.[88,141]

18.6.4 Possible Interactions with Herbs and other Dietary Supplements

- Used in conjunction with vitamin and mineral supplements, long-term psyllium use may reduce absorption of nutrients, including calcium, iron, zinc, and vitamin B12.[141]

18.6.5 Possible Interactions with Diseases or Conditions

- Type 2 (non-insulin-dependent) diabetes
- Some GI conditions

• Kidney dysfunction: Raw seeds contain a potentially nephrotoxic agent (removed in most commercial sources)

• Phenylketonuria: "Sugar-free" commercial sources often contain aspartame.

18.6.6 Typical Dosage

• **Oral:** Adult dose is 3.5 g of blonde psyllium husk 3-5 times daily; Children's (6-12 years) dose is half the adult dose. For hypercholesterolemia: FDA evaluated studies used 10.2 g of psyllium seed husk (about 7 g of soluble fiber) daily.[141] When used as part of a synergistic gastrointestinal formula: 300 mg of dried herb, 3 times per day.

Note: Adequate fluid intake is necessary: A minimum of 240 mL per 5.1 g or less of psyllium husk.[141]

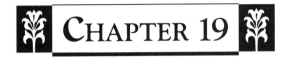

CHAPTER 19

ALFALFA
Medicago sativa

BARLEY GRASS
Hordeum vulgare

BUCKWHEAT
Fagopyrum esculentum

19

⇒⟩⟩⧽|⧽⟨⟨⇐

ALFALFA
Medicago sativa

BARLEY GRASS
Hordeum vulgare

BUCKWHEAT
Fagopyrum esculentum

19.1 Description and Medical History

Barley grass and **alfalfa** are bioavailable sources of protein and contain a wide array of vitamins, minerals, and enzymes that are crucial for maintaining health. Green young barley leaves have been reported to have numerous health properties, including:

- anti-aging[114,217]
- anti-carcinogenic[114,217]
- anti-diabetic[114,217]
- anti-atherosclerotic[114,217]

A potent flavonoid antioxidant, 2"-O-glycosylisovitexin (2O-GIV), was isolated as the putative active agent for these effects. Alfalfa contains a significant amount of **vitamin K** and

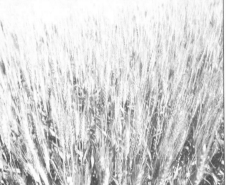

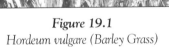
Figure 19.1
Hordeum vulgare (Barley Grass)

coumesterol, which function synergistically to maintain proper bone density.[73] Alfalfa also contains **chlorophyll**, which has been shown to protect against environmental mutagens and carcinogens.[16,119]

Buckwheat contains **inositol**, methionine, lysine, and cysteine.[171] Buckwheat also contains **rutin** and **quercitin**, two antioxidants that offer cellular protection against oxidative damage,[277,297] and the seeds contain potent proanthocyanidin antioxidants.[264]

19.2 Known Medicinal Constituents

19.2.1 Alfalfa

- Vitamins: A, C, E, and K4
- Minerals: calcium, potassium, phosphorous, and iron
- Carotinoids
- Isoflavonoids: including formononetin, genistein, and daidzein [See 17. *Trifolium pratense* (Red Clover)]
- Coumestans: coumestrol, lucernol, sativol, and trifoliol
- Triterpene saponins

19.2.2 Barley Grass

- Polysaccharides (50% of seeds): chiefly starch and fructans, including β-glucan
- Mono- and oligosaccharides: saccharose, raffinose, glucose, and fructose
- Proteins (10% of seeds): prolamines, albumins, and globulins
- Vitamins: E, nicotinic acid, pantothenic acid, B6, B2, and folic acid
- Hydroxycoumarins (stalks only):
  including umbelliferone, scopoletin, herniarin, and aesculetin (in sprouts)
- Amines: hordenine (dimethyl tyramine) and tyramine

19.2.3 Buckwheat

- Flavonoids: rutin (up to 8% in leaves) and quercitin[141]
- Anthracene derivatives (naphthadianthrones): fagopyrine (0.01%) and protofagopyrine[141]

19.3 Indications for Use

19.3.1 Alfalfa

- Vitamin and mineral deficiency[141]

- Hypercholesterolemia
- Diuretic for kidney, bladder, and prostate conditions[141]
- Folk medicine: Diabetes and thyroid conditions[141]

19.3.2 Barley Grass

- Stomach upset, diarrhea, gastritis, or inflammatory bowel conditions
- Hypercholesterolemia
- Hyperglycemia
- Poor circulation and bronchoconstriction

19.3.3 Buckwheat

- Edema and poor venous tone[141]
- Venous stasis, varicose veins, and arterial sclerosis (folk medicine)[141]
- Skin and liver diseases with itching and headache (homeopathic use)[141]

19.4 Mechanisms of Action

19.4.1 Alfalfa

- Alfalfa is high in chlorophyll, a molecule that appears to inhibit the mutagenicity of some carcinogens.[119,384] It is thought that chlorophylls and their derivatives can form molecular complexes with toxins, inactivating them by preventing their binding to DNA and cellular receptors.[56,63,119,283] Chlorophyll may also non-specifically inhibit cytochrome P450 activity, reducing Phase I molecular processes that may lead to carcinogen activation.[384]

- The saponins found in alfalfa leaves act on the cardiovascular, nervous, and digestive systems.[141] They appear to decrease plasma cholesterol without changing HDL cholesterol levels. The constituents in alfalfa may decrease cholesterol absorption and increase the excretion of bile acids and neutral steroids.

- Alfalfa contains phytoestrogens which may have estrogenic properties.

19.4.2 Barley Grass

- Flavonoids in barley grass possess strong antioxidant activity inhibiting lipid peroxidation.[217]

- The fiber content of barley is responsible for the blood cholesterol and glucose-lowering activity of barley.[141] β-glucans in barley probably reduce appetite by slowing gastric emptying and stabilizing blood sugar.

- Barley contains hordenine, a sympathomimetic amine that stimulates peripheral blood circulation and bronchodilation.[141]

19.4.3 Buckwheat

- Rutin is responsible for the antiedematic activity of buckwheat.[141] Very little information is available on the mechanisms of action of buckwheat.

19.5 Research

19.5.1 Chlorophyll and Cancer

Alfalfa and other green foods are rich in chlorophyll. Studies indicate that chlorophyll and its derivatives have potential chemoprotective and anticarcinogenic effects in animals and humans,[56,119,283,384] though the mechanism is not entirely clear.

Researchers[384] propose that chlorophyll mainly acts by inhibiting the cytochrome P450 enzymatic pathway that is responsible for the activation of some carcinogens. The experimenters examined the *in vitro* effects of chlorophyllin, the sodium/copper derivative of chlorophyll, on the P450 activity of rat and human liver microsomes. Table 19.1 shows the loss of CYP450 activity for all the rat and human liver enzyme systems assayed in this study. The inhibition was non-specific and NADPH-dependent.

19.5.2 Barley Grass and Atherosclerosis

Young barley leaves contain 2"-O-glycosylisovitexin (2O-GIV), a flavonoid molecule that may reduce the risk of atherosclerosis by inhibiting the peroxidation of lipids.[217] Using low density lipoprotein (LDL) and blood plasma from a horse, these researchers examined the antioxidative activity of 2O-GIV and found that the amount of acetaldehyde (a biproduct of LDL peroxidation) produced was lower in the presence of 2O-GIV. Furthermore, the putative inhibition of peroxidation was dose dependent for 2O-GIV and ferulic acid, a known antioxidant (Figure 19.2) In blood plasma, 2O-GIV was nearly identical to the antiatherosclerotic drug probucol in reducing acetaldehyde production in this model (data not shown). Identical amounts (0.3μmol) of 2O-GIV and probucol inhibited acetaldehyde formation by 89% and 94%, respectively.

Enzymatic activity (CYP450)	Microsome sample	Rate (nmol product/ min/mg protein)	% inhibition of activity (μM chlorophyllin)				
			0	10	20	50	100
Human liver microsomes							
1A2	HL108	2.4×10^{-3}	0	54	82	>99	>99
2A6	HL115	2.3	0	56	70	88	98
2E1	HL99	1.5	0	35	60	96	>99
2A6, 1A2, 2B6, 2F1	HL115	7.8×10^{-1}	0	58	78	84	97
3A4, 1A2, 2C8/9/10	HL110	1.4×10^{-1}	0	45	60	89	94
3A4	HL110	4.0	0	40	70	87	95
3A4, 2B6	HL108	2.6×10^{-3}	0	65	85	>99	>99
Rat liver microsomes							
1A	Untreated	1.0×10^{-1}	0	36	68	82	95
2B1/2	Untreated	3.5×10^{-1}	0	34	74	96	>99
2E1	Pyridine treated	1.6×10^{2}	0	56	75	90	94

Table 19.1
Inhibition of CYP450 activity by chlorophyllin in human and rat liver microsomes[384]

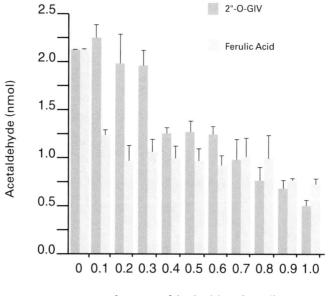

Figure 19.2

Inhibitory effect of 2O-GIV and ferulic acid on LDL oxidation in the horse; adapted from Miyake et al.[217]

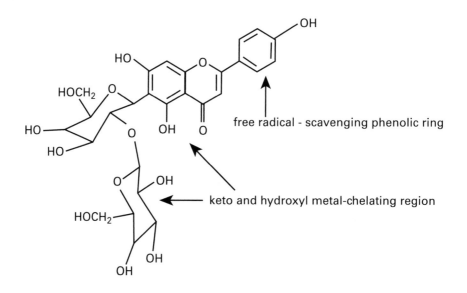

Figure 19.3

The 2O-GIV molecule has free radical-scavenging phenolic regions and metal-chelating keto- and hydroxyl-groups; adapted from Miyake et al.[217]

It is believed that 2O-GIV acts as an antioxidant both by chelating metal ions and by scavenging free radicals, based on the putative reactive regions of the molecule.

There appeared to be a synergistic effect between 2O-GIV and vitamin C in preventing oxidative acetaldehyde formation in the blood plasma of the horse.[217] While 2O-GIV was a more potent antioxidant than vitamin C in the model used, the combination of the two substances had a significantly greater effect than either one alone (Figure 19.4).

19.5.3 Buckwheat and Cancer

Rutin and quercetin are found in large amounts in buckwheat and several other foods such as apples. These putative chemopreventive molecules, among others, were assessed by Wargovich et al[361] for their ability to prevent aberrant crypt foci development in the colons of rats. When added as purified compounds to the diet of rats, both rutin and quercetin caused

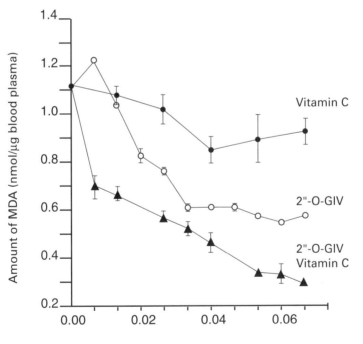

Figure 19.4
Synergistic antioxidative activities of 2O-GIV and vitamin C in blood plasma of the horse; adapted from Miyake et al.[217]

significant dose-dependent reductions in the post-initiation occurrence of aberrant crypts in colons of the rats (Table 19.2). It is important to note that the compounds were administered post-initiation (by azoxymethane) when aberrant crypt foci had already progressed to multiple crypt clusters. Thus, the results indicate an inhibition of further outgrowth of aberrant crypts into multiple crypt clusters. As aberrant crypts are thought to be a precursor of colon cancer in both animals and humans,[273,321] this result suggests a good potential for the inhibition of colon cancer development due to these molecules.

Agent	Dose (g/kg diet)	Aberrant crypts/colon	
		Mean±SEM	% of control
Quercetin	0	133±4	100
	15	74±5	56[a]
	30	70±5	53[a]
Rutin	0	133±4	100
	15	81±6	61[a]
	30	41±3	31[a]
[a] $p < 0.05$			

Table 19.2
Effect of rutin and quercetin on AOM-induced aberrant crypt foci in the rat colon during the post-initiation phase of carcinogenesis.[361]

19.5.4 Buckwheat, Cholesterol, and Gall Bladder Function

Tomotake et al[335] examined the effect of buckwheat protein on serum and liver cholesterol levels in Golden Syrian hamsters fed a cholesterol diet (5g/kg cholesterol). The hamster was used as an animal model because its cholesterol and bile acid metabolism is similar in several ways to that of humans. In the gall bladder, cholesterol is dissolved in bile acids and phospholipids. If the biliary concentration of cholesterol exceeds the amount of bile acid needed to dissolve it, gallstones can develop.

Hamsters were divided into three groups of eight and each group was fed on a cholesterol diet with one of the following sources of protein:

- Casein
- Soy protein
- Buckwheat protein

Although the weight gain of the rats fed soy protein was significantly higher than the other two groups, the food consumption of the buckwheat group was significantly higher than the casein and soy groups. Plasma total cholesterol was significantly lower in the buckwheat group than the other two with a higher ratio of HDL to total cholesterol. Liver cholesterol was markedly lower in the buckwheat group as well. While none of the buckwheat protein-fed hamsters developed gallstones, two of the hamsters fed soy protein and all eight of the hamsters fed casein had visible gallstones. The concentration and molar percentage of cholesterol in bile was significantly lower while bile acids were slightly elevated in the buckwheat protein group relative to the casein-fed group. Soy protein had a similar but significantly weaker effect to buckwheat protein on bile cholesterol concentration. The buckwheat protein diet caused a significant increase in the fecal excretion of cholesterol and neutral steroids. In addition to buckwheat's favorable effects on cholesterol metabolism and gallstone formation, *the findings of this research study also provide evidence that supports the use of buckwheat as a superior protein source for growth, in comparison to soy.* The data are summarized in Table 19.3.

19.6 Overview

These clinical results coupled with the results of earlier trials strongly suggest that green vegetables such as **alfalfa, barley grass, and buckwheat:**

- Regulate Phase I enzymatic detoxification mechanisms
- Inhibit colon cancer development
- Reduce the risk of atherosclerosis

19.6.1 Contraindications

Alfalfa

- None known

	Casein diet	Soy protein diet	Buckwheat protein diet
Gallstones	8/8	2/8	0/8
Plasma lipids			
Total cholesterol (mmol/L)	6.88 ± 0.32^a	6.21 ± 0.28^a	5.02 ± 0.22^b
HDL cholesterol (mmol/L)	2.43 ± 0.09^a	2.68 ± 0.12^a	2.15 ± 0.06^b
Triglycerides (mmol/L)	10.75 ± 1.63^a	6.21 ± 0.44^b	4.89 ± 0.40^b
Phospholipids (mmol/L)	7.19 ± 0.35^a	7.06 ± 0.48^a	4.85 ± 0.18^b
Liver lipids			
Cholesterol (μmol/g)	49.5 ± 3.3^a	45.4 ± 4.0^a	23.5 ± 2.1^b
Triglycerides (μmol/g)	5.62 ± 0.33	5.24 ± 0.41	4.69 ± 0.28
Phospholipids (μmol/g)	9.21 ± 0.71	8.13 ± 0.72	7.79 ± 0.78
Biliary lipids			
Cholesterol (mmol/L)	22.1 ± 2.4^a	10.4 ± 1.1^b	4.0 ± 0.2^c
Cholesterol (mol/100 mol lipids)	13.9 ± 1.4^a	8.3 ± 0.5^b	3.5 ± 0.4^c
Phospholipids (mmol/L)	25.2 ± 2.8^a	17.4 ± 1.5^b	7.7 ± 0.5^c
Phospholipids (mol/100 mol lipids)	15.3 ± 1.0^a	14.1 ± 0.5^a	6.5 ± 0.4^b
Bile acids (mmol/L)	116.4 ± 9.9	95.5 ± 6.9	109.0 ± 9.0
Bile acids (mol/100 mol lipids)	70.9 ± 1.2^c	77.6 ± 0.8^b	90.0 ± 0.7^a
Within a row, means with the same superscript are not significantly different ($p < 0.05$).			

Table 19.3
*Serum, liver, and gall bladder lipid parameters in hamsters fed a cholesterol diet
containing casein, soy protein, or buckwheat protein. Adapted from Tomotake et al.[335]*

Barley Grass

- Allergic sensitivity to barley[141]
- Celiac disease (gluten sensitivity)[141]

Buckwheat

- None known

19.6.2 Side Effects

Alfalfa

- None known

Barley Grass

- Anaphylaxis in sensitive individuals[141]

Buckwheat

- None known

19.6.3 Possible Interactions with Drugs

Alfalfa

- Alfalfa contains vitamin K, an essential blood coagulation factor that may, in high quantities, increase the risk of clotting in people taking anticoagulant drugs.[141]
- In theory, large amounts of alfalfa may interfere with hormone replacement therapy or oral contraceptives via competition of phytoestrogens for sex hormone receptors.[47,141]
- Excessive doses of alfalfa may potentiate chlorpromazine-induced photosensitivity.[36]

Barley Grass

- Hordenine content may potentiate effect of sympathomimetic drugs[141]

Buckwheat

- None known

19.6.4 Possible Interactions with Herbs and other Dietary Supplements

Alfalfa

- The saponins in alfalfa may interfere with absorption or activity of vitamin E.[141]

19.6.5 Possible Interactions with Diseases or Conditions

Alfalfa

- Consumption of seeds, but not stems/leaves, might reactivate latent systemic lupus erythematosus (SLE).[36]

- The phytoestrogens found in alfalfa may interact with estrogen sensitive diseases or conditions.[141]

Barley grass

- Barley gluten content may exacerbate celiac disease.[141]

Buckwheat

- None known

19.6.6 Typical Dosage

Alfalfa

- Variable

- When used as part of a synergistic gastrointestinal formula: 200 mg of dried herb, 3 times per day.

Barley grass

- 450 mg – 900 mg dried grass

- When used as part of a synergistic gastrointestinal formula: 300 mg of dried grass, 3 times per day.

Buckwheat

- Orally as drops, tablets, and in teas. Dosage variable

- When used as part of a synergistic gastrointestinal formula: 300 mg of dried herb, 3 times per day.

Monographs
Barley Grass
Alfalfa Buckwheat

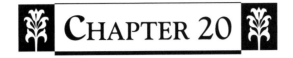

CHAPTER 20

BRUSSELS SPROUTS   BROCCOLI   KALE

Brassica spp.

20
❧

BRUSSELS SPROUTS BROCCOLI KALE

Brassica spp.

20.1 Description and Medical History

Brussels sprouts, broccoli, and kale are members of the Brassicaceae plant family. This family contains numerous anticarcinogenic and detoxifying nutrients.[26,238] **Glucosinolate compounds** are a particular group of phytonutrients found in brassicas that are of great importance with respect to cancer and the liver detoxification system. The medicinal properties of glucosinolates are noted in the writings of Pythagoras and Hippocrates and at least 20 different compounds were identified by the 1980s.[190] All cruciferous vegetables are believed to contain glucosinolates, but Brussels sprouts and broccoli have some of the highest levels.

The glucosinolates found in whole foods break down into indoles, isothiocyanates, and other important compounds when ingested. **Sulforaphane** and **sinigrin** isothiocyanate are two isothiocyanates that protect against, and oftentimes reduce, the severity of lung, colon, stomach, liver, and breast cancers.[111] Sulforaphane supports the enzymatic activity that takes place in Phase I liver detoxification and assists the liver in carrying out the Phase II conjugation pathways. Sinigrin isothiocyanate complements the activity of sulforaphane by also stimulating the Phase II detoxification system.

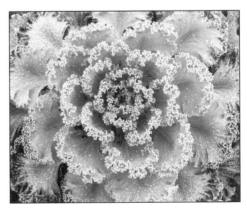

Figure 20.1
Kale (member of the Brassica family)

In addition to supporting the liver detoxification system, sinigrin isothiocyanate stimulates apoptosis, a process that naturally causes a damaged cell to fragment into membrane-bound particles that are then eliminated by phagocytosis. Kale is also a potent source of lutein and zeaxanthin, the only two carotenoids that are found in the eye. These carotenoids reduce oxidative damage to the eyes, preventing and in some cases reducing, the damaging effects of free radicals in the eyes.[323]

Indole-3-carbinol is an indole derivative found in most brassica species. *In vivo*, most studies report a chemoprotective role for this compound.[64,309] Brassicas also are low in fat, low in energy, and are potent sources of vitamins, minerals, fiber, and phytochemicals, all of which have been linked to cancer prevention[85,236] The isothiocyanate phytochemicals in brassica vegetables primarily induce Phase II detoxification, conjugating and polarizing toxins for better excretability.[261]

In people under 55 years of age, cruciferous vegetable intake is inversely correlated with colon cancer incidence and among smokers the chemoprotective benefits of brassica consumption were even better.[303,356] Broccoli has shown the strongest correlations. Van Poppel et al[346] examined six cohort studies and 74 case control studies that supported an inverse correlation between brassica consumption and cancer risk. The association was found to be most consistent for lung, stomach, colon, and rectal cancers, and least consistent for prostatic, endometrial, and ovarian cancers. In studies examining total vegetable consumption an inverse association with cancer risk is also found with the brassicas showing the strongest effects as a subgroup.[356]

In brassicas, there appears to be no net synthesis of Phase II inducers after sprouting and their concentration decreases as the plant grows.[236] As a result, brassica sprouts may contain 10-100 times the Phase II induction activity of mature plants. Indeed, extracts of broccoli sprouts have been shown to be more efficient at inhibiting rat tumorigenesis than extracts of mature plants.[85] Conversely, mature broccoli contains significant amounts of indole compounds not found in sprouts that induce both Phase I and II detoxification enzymes.[236]

20.2 Research

20.2.1 Brassicas and Liver Detoxification

Researchers[309] examined the effects of a mixture of glucosinolate breakdown products from Brussels sprouts on the induction of liver detoxification enzymes in rats. The mixture (full strength, 60%, and 20%) elevated levels of cytochrome P450 1A (CYP1A), glutathione-S-transferase (GST), quinone reductase (QR), glutathione reductase (GR), and glutathione (GSH) in a dose dependant manner, supporting the hypothesis that glucosinolates found in green vegetables are important in the regulation of hepatic detoxification (Table 20.1).

The following Brussels sprout glucosinolate breakdown products and amounts were used in the mixture fed to the rats:

- Indole-3-carbinol (I3C; 56 mg/kg)
- Iberin (38 mg/kg)
- Phenylethylisothiocyanate (PEITC; 0.1 mg/kg)
- Cyanohydroxybutene (crambene; 50 mg/kg)

The amounts reflect the proportionate amounts of each glucosinolate compound found in Brussels sprouts standardized to 50 mg crambene/kg (induces glutathione without toxic effects).

Treatment	CYP 1A[a]	GST[b]	QR[c]	GR[d]	GSH[e]
Undiluted mixture					
100% mix	1378.0±54.1*	1343.4±79.8*	185.9±10.8*	54.3±3.22*	5.53±0.16
Control	124.2±7.3	541.0±41.4	30.0±2.4	30.6±0.85	2.71±0.12
Pair-fed	84.8±7.8	511.0±35.9	32.5±4.8	28.2±1.51	2.77±0.06
Diluted Mixture					
60% mix	606.8±47.1*	728.5±52.5*	168.7±21.1*	44.8±2.2*	2.82±1.06
20% mix	211.5±22.4*	499.0±34.0*	109.2±8.4*	37.5±0.86*	2.46±0.30
Control	60.9±6.0	369.5±32.0	70.7±12.0	30.6±0.88	3.24±0.44
Pair-fed	50.2±3.9	421.2±37.1	49.7±5.7	30.4±0.86	3.36±0.32

In addition to an antioxidant-free diet, rats were fed the glucosinolate mixture by lavage 12 hours after daily feeding.

[a] Ethoxyresorufin dealkylation (pmol/min/mg microsomal protein) [b] CDNB conjugate formation (nm/min/mg cytosolic protein)
[c] DCPP reduced (nm/min/mg cytosolic protein) [d] NADPH oxidized (nm/min/mg cytosolic protein) [e] GSH (μmol/gm liver weight)

* Significantly different from control (p<0.05)

Table 20.1

*Dose-dependent induction of Phase II detoxification molecules in response to
ingestion of a mixture of Brussels sprout glucosinolate breakdown products.*[309]

It is important to note that in this study the individual glucosinolate breakdown products were also tested. While indole-3-carbinol (I3C) was the only glucosinolate in the mixture to significantly increase enzyme activity, the glucosinolate mixture containing I3C was considerably more effective, supporting a synergistic mechanism of action between the compounds. This suggests that bioactive molecules ingested as part of a complete nutritional regimen may be considerably more effective than the isolated active principles used alone.

Preliminary data suggest that a commercially available complex of vacuum dried organic alfalfa, buckwheat, Brussels sprouts, barley grass, and kale (SP GreenFood®, Standard Process, Inc.) induces significant increases in quinone reductase activity in both human and mouse hepatoma cell lines (Dr. Elizabeth Jeffery, University of Illinois-Urbana/Champagne, personal communication).

Isothiocyanates have also been shown to act as anticarcinogens by inducing detoxification of environmental mutagens.[190] Sulforaphane blocked 7,12-dimethylbenz(a)-anthracene-induced mammary tumors in rats[390] and broccoli extract was a potent inducer of detoxification enzymes in a mouse hepatoma cell assay, probably due to sulforaphane as well.[389]

Fifty percent of people completely lack the glutathione-S-transferase M1 (GSTM1) enzyme due to a homozygous gene deletion. This enzyme is responsible for the rapid conjugation of isothiocyanates to glutathione for excretion (Phase II). Lin et al[190] hypothesized that people with this mutation would maintain higher levels of isothiocyanates in the body due to decreased excretion and should show a lower incidence of colorectal adenomas, the precursors of colorectal cancer, if isothiocyanates are indeed anticarcinogenic. The researchers found that broccoli and kale, but not cabbage, cauliflower, or Brussels sprouts, were significantly associated with lower prevalence of colorectal carcinomas in a sample of nearly a thousand people (459 adenoma cases and 507 controls sampled from patients undergoing cancer sigmoidoscopy screening in southern California). The presence of the GSTM1 null genotype alone did not significantly correlate with the occurrence of colorectal carcinoma. However, the GSTM1 null genotype did correlate with a significant reduction of incidence of colorectal carcinoma when it was covaried with broccoli and total cruciferous vegetable consumption (p=0.001 and p=0.02, respectively). The lowest incidence of colorectal carcinoma occurred in GSTM1 null individuals in the highest quartile of broccoli consumption, supporting the hypothesis that isothiocyanates in crucifers may be excreted more slowly in urine in GSTM1 individuals. However, neither urinary nor serum isothiocyanate measurements were taken in the subjects, so other mechanisms cannot be ruled out. It is clear from the body of research available that consumption of higher levels of cruciferous vegetables is indicated for reducing the risk of some cancers.

20.2.2 Brassicas and Cancer

Verhoeven et al[350] examined the results of seven cohort studies and 87 case-control studies on the association between brassica vegetable consumption and cancer risk. In five of the cohort studies, brassica consumption correlated inversely with the risk of certain cancers. The specific findings are summarized in Table 20.2.

Of the 87 case-control studies, 68 (78%) found a lower cancer risk associated with consumption of brassica vegetables, although not all were significant and some applied to only one sex. The number of case-control studies in which at least one significant inverse relationship between brassicas and cancer risk was found is shown in Table 20.3.

Although the percentage of case-control studies showing a significant inverse relationship between brassica consumption and cancer risk is less than half in most cases, bear in mind that other variables known and unknown undoubtedly play a role in the relationship. Furthermore, only one study showed a positive correlation, suggesting that the inverse relationship between brassica consumption and cancer is real and not simply an artifact of chance.

Study population	Follow-up	Cancer type	Brassica vegetable	Variables adjusted for
13,785 men and 2,928 women in Norway[172]	11.5 years (113 cancer cases)	Lung	Cabbage, cauliflower, and rutabaga	Age, smoking, region, urban/rural
1,271 elderly people in Massachusetts[59]	5 years (42 cancer deaths)	All types	Broccoli	Age
8,006 men of Japanese ancestry in Hawaii[57]	18 years (111 cancer cases)	Stomach	All brassicas	Age, current smoking status
41,837 postmenopausal women in Iowa[314]	4 years (138 cancer cases)	Lung	Broccoli Cabbage, broccoli,	Age, energy intake, smoking
1,090 oral and pharyngeal cancer patients in the U.S.[65]	5 years (80 cases of second primary cancer)	Varied	Brussels sprouts, and coleslaw	Age, index tumor stage, smoking, drinking, energy intake

Table 20.2
Prospective cohort studies showing a significant inverse relationship between consumption of brassica vegetables and cancer risk (five studies out of seven).[350]

Because DNA damage is considered a pathogenic event in the initiation of many cancers,[26] the urinary excretion of biomarkers of DNA damage serves as an potential indicator of cancer risk. An abundant and potentially mutagenic lesion caused by oxidative DNA damage is the incorporation of 8-oxo-7,8-dihydro-2'-deoxyguanosine (8-oxodG) adducts into the DNA strand.[349] Normal DNA repair mechanisms excise 8-oxodG, which is excreted unchanged and independent of diet in the urine. Thus, the relative rate of excretion represents the integrated rate of oxidative DNA damage in the body.

Verhagen's group investigated the hypothesis that dietary cruciferous vegetables result in a reduction of oxidative DNA damage in healthy, male, non-smoking humans. Ten volunteers consumed a diet containing 300g of cooked, non-cruciferous vegetables (endive, French beans, peas, beets, fava beans, chicory and assorted other legumes and vegetables) per meal during a three week run-in period. During the subsequent three week intervention period, five of the volunteers continued on this diet (control group) while five others began consuming 300 g of cooked Brussels sprouts at the expense of 300g of a glucosinolate-free vegetable. 24-hour urine samples were collected at the end of the run-in and intervention periods. The Brussels sprouts caused no adverse effects as measured by several clinico-chemical parameters for liver, renal, thyroid, and blood-coagulation functions. During the run-in period, there was no difference in 8-oxodG excretion between the sprouts and cruciferous vegetable-free groups. Within the control group, there was no significant change in excretion between the run-in and the intervention period. By contrast, the 8-oxodG excretion decreased by 28% in the Brussels sprouts group during the intervention period.

Cancer type	Total Number of Studies	Number of studies showing a significant inverse association	Number of studies showing a significant positive association
Colon	15	6 (40%)	0
Stomach	11	5 (45%)	1 (9%)
Rectum	10	4 (40%)	0
Lung	9	6 (67%)	0

Table 20.3
Case-control studies showing a significant relationship between cancer risk and consumption of brassica vegetables by cancer type (positive and negative correlations).[350]

20.3 Overview

These clinical results coupled with the results of earlier trials strongly suggest that **Brassicas:**

- Detoxify by upregulating detoxification enzymes
- Prevent oxidative cell and DNA damage
- Are chemoprotective against numerous types of cancer

Monographs
Brussels Sprouts
Broccoli Kale

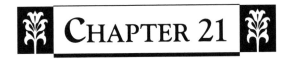
CHOLINE

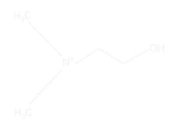

21

--->>>|<<<---

CHOLINE

21.1 Description and Medical History

Choline is a precursor of the neurotransmitter acetylcholine and is also involved in methyl group metabolism and lipid transport.[46,141] It is an essential structural component of biological membranes and plasma lipoproteins. Thus, it is not surprising that it plays a major role in lipid metabolism. It has been shown to be essential for normal liver function in humans, rats, hamsters, guinea pigs, pigs, dogs, monkeys, trout, quail, and chicken.[388] Choline is a lipotropic agent involved in lipid mobilization and the removal of excess fat from the liver.[110,141,387] It is intimately involved in cellular signal transduction cascades regulating cell transport, metabolism, gene expression, and growth.[46]

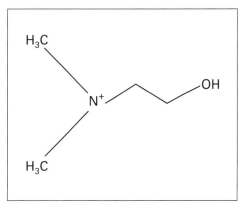

Choline is manufactured naturally by the body, however research suggests that choline is an essential dietary nutrient[37,387] considered to be a component of the vitamin B complex. Choline is readily available in numerous foods, including

Figure 21.1
Molecular structure of Choline

meats, fish, nuts, beans, peas, and eggs. Liver, kidney, and brain tissues also have a high choline content.[141] Choline is a constituent of phosphatidylcholine, which is a component of lecithin.[141]

Choline deficiency causes liver cancer in rat models as a result of the generation of free radicals, DNA alterations, and liver cell death.[103] Consumption of a choline deficient diet impairs liver antioxidant defenses in rats leading to lipid peroxidation.[110] Choline deficiency causes steatosis (fatty liver) and early signs of liver dysfunction in both animals and humans.[37,110,298,387] Thus, it appears to be important for balanced liver function. In conjunction, these findings suggest choline deficiency predisposes fatty liver tissue to oxidative damage and cancer. Hence, choline can be considered an antioxidant that is hepatoprotective.

21.2 Indications for Use

- Liver carcinogenesis
- Fatty liver
- Choline insufficiency

21.3 Mechanisms of Action

Because choline is involved in many biochemical pathways in the body, it is difficult to define a particular mode of action for the nutrient. However, the research does show several key mechanisms by which the nutrient functions in the liver:

- Choline deficiency lessens the ability of key tissues, such as liver and brain to properly utilize folate.[14] Folate plays a major role in intracellular metabolism.[141] It is involved in DNA synthesis and can protect and reduce replication errors via methylation of DNA.[196,302] This has implications for cancer prevention. Folate also increases the conversion of homocysteine to methionine, lowering elevated homocysteine levels that have been linked to heart disease.[55,176,352] Thus, choline acts indirectly via its effect on folate metabolism.

- Humans fed parenterally show decreased plasma choline concentrations and develop liver dysfunction similar to that seen in choline-deficient animals.[388] Choline supplementation alleviates the condition. In choline deficient experimental animals, fatty liver occurs because phosphatidylcholine synthesis is required for VLDL cholesterol secretion by the liver. The accumulation of lipids in the liver may explain the observation that choline-deficient rats spontaneously develop hepatocarcinoma. Choline deficiency was associated with the accumulation of 1,2-diacylglycerol, an activator of the signal transduction molecule protein kinase C.[388] Additionally, carbohydrate loading, a condition that enhances hepatic triglyceride synthesis, increases the body's requirement for choline to facilitate triglyceride export from the liver. Thus, starchy, high calorie diets with insufficient choline probably exacerbate the fatty liver condition.

Note: Interestingly, serum cholesterol actually drops in humans fed a choline deficient diet as a result of decreased secretion of VLDL by the liver.[387]

• **Deficiency in dietary choline is sufficient to trigger carcinogenesis in animals without exposure to any known carcinogens.**[51,101] Some of the acute effects of a choline deficient diet are related to generation of free radicals and subsequent lipid peroxidation, especially in liver cell membranes.[251] An antioxidant, AD5, was found to be very effective in preventing nuclear lipid peroxidation, DNA damage, and cell death induced by a choline deficient diet in rats.[102] However, it had little effect on the accumulation of triglycerides, which require VLDL cholesterol packaging to be removed from the liver.[388] Thus, oxygen free radicals might be an important component in the early events of liver carcinogenesis induced by a choline deficient diet. In addition, choline deficiency can increase the activity of protein

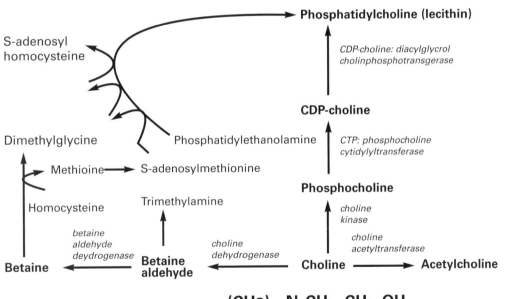

Figure 21.1

Choline metabolism: Choline is a precursor of several biologically important molecules, including lecithin (a cellular membrane constituent), betaine (a methyl donor and putative antioxidant), and acetylcholine (a neurotransmitter).

kinase C (PKC) involved in control of gene expression, cell division, and differentiation.[388] Oncogenes, thought to trigger cell division in cancerous cells, demonstrate over expression in the liver and tumor tissues of choline deficient mice and rats.[52,132]

• Choline is oxidized in the body to form betaine, an important antioxidant and methyl donor in biochemical reactions, particularly the conversion of homocysteine to methionine.[17,388]

21.4 Research

21.4.1 Choline and Liver Carcinogenesis

Male Fischer 344 rats fed a choline-methionine deficient (CMD) diet for 13-24 months developed putative pre-neoplastic hepatocyte nodules in 100% of cases and hepatocellular carcinoma in 51% of cases compared to zero incidence in controls fed the same diet supplemented with 0.8% choline chloride.[101] This effect was observed in the absence of any known exogenous or endogenous carcinogens. In addition, four rats fed the CMD diet developed metastases to the lungs (Table 21.1).

Note: Methionine deficiency is required for choline deficiency to prevent de novo choline synthesis from methionine in the body.

Body weights did not differ among animals up to 72 weeks, although animals with cancer at autopsy showed loss of weight 2-4 weeks prior to sacrifice.

Diet	Time span (months)	N	No. of animals with hepatocyte nodules	No. of animals with hepatocellular carcinoma	No. of animals with metastasis to the lung
CMD	13-24*	45	45 (100%)	23 (51%)	4 (17%)
Control		45	0	0	–
* First cancer detected at 13 months exposure to the CMD diet					

Table 21.1
Effects of a choline-methionine deficient diet on the occurrence of liver cancer in rats.[101]

Researchers[276] showed that a choline deficient diet resulted in significant DNA damage in the liver of rats, even when fed for as few as three days. The damage was repairable inasmuch as supplementation of the diet with choline caused a disappearance of accumulated damage. The authors suggest that the induction of DNA damage by choline deficiency may be an important early initiation event in liver carcinogenesis. Lipid peroxidation due to the accumulation of lipids in the liver has been proposed as a possible mechanism in liver cancer induced by choline deficiency.[275]

21.4.2 Choline and Liver Lipid Peroxidation

A choline and methionine deficient diet induced lipid peroxidation in the purified nuclear fraction of rat liver within one day of exposure.[275] No such change was observed in rats fed the same diet supplemented with 1.45g/100 g choline bitartrate. This study was the first to show lipid peroxidation in the nuclear fraction of liver cells and they observed no lipid peroxidation in mitochondria or microsomes as is seen with CCl_4 hepatotoxicity. This provides a reasonable explanation for the DNA damage observed in choline deficiency[276] and may provide a mechanism for the carcinogenesis induced by this diet. Several chemical carcinogens and tumor promoting factors also are known to generate free radicals that damage DNA.[80,301]

21.5   Overview

These clinical results coupled with the results of earlier trials strongly suggest that **choline:**

- Prevents development of "fatty liver"
- Prevents development of liver steatosis
- Protects the liver against cancer induced by choline deficiency
- Protects DNA from putative oxidative damage
- May be cardioprotective

21.5.1 Contraindications

- None known

21.5.2 Side Effects

Although side effects are rare, they can include:

- Sweating
- Gastrointestinal distress
- Vomiting
- Diarrhea (with large doses)

Most adults can tolerate up to 20 g of choline per day and some as much as 30g. Choline can cause a "fishy" body odor in some people.[141]

21.5.3 Possible Interactions with Drugs

- None known

21.5.4 Possible Interactions with Herbs and other Dietary Supplements

- Insufficient reliable information

21.5.5 Possible interactions with Diseases or Conditions

- None known

21.5.6 Typical Dosage

- The average diet supplies 200-600 mg of choline per day. 550 mg per day is recommended for males and lactating females. Most women need 425-450 mg per day. Most children require 200-375 mg per day, depending on age. Maximum daily dosages should not exceed 1-2 g for children and 3-3.5 g for adults. When used as part of a synergistic detoxification formula: 100 mg, 3 times per day.

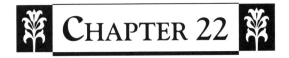

CHAPTER 22

INOSITOL

22

INOSITOL

22.1 Description and Medical History

Inositol, sometimes called myoinositol, is an isomer of glucose that exists in numerous biological forms.[129] Most commonly it is found in its free form, in inositol phospholipids, or as phytic acid (inositol hexaphosphate). Phytic acid (phytate) is the common form in plant foodstuffs, such as cereals, fruits, and vegetables. The gut enzyme phytase hydrolyzes phytate into free inositol and intermediary mono-, di-, tri, tetra-, and pentaphosphate esters of inositol. The inositol and phosphorous released is absorbed mainly in the small intestine.

Endogenous inositol is a major component of cell membrane phospholipids.[141] It is weakly lipotropic in its ability to move fat out of liver and intestinal cells.[141]

Inositol deficiency in animals causes an accumulation of triglycerides in the liver and intestinal lipodystrophy.[129] Altered metabolism of inositol has been documented in patients with diabetes mellitus, chronic renal failure, galactosemia, psychiatric disease and multiple sclerosis.[129]

Although it has not been demonstrated in humans, preliminary research suggests that inositol hexaphosphate (IP6; phytate) can lower serum cholesterol and triglyceride levels.[140]

Myoinositol and IP6 decrease dietary sucrose-induced rises in hepatic lipids and lipogenic enzymes.[156]

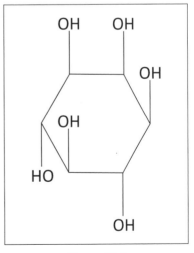

Figure 22.1
Molecular structure of Inositol

22.2 Indications for Use

- Elevated triglycerides
- Fatty liver
- Tumorigenesis

22.3 Possible Mechanisms of Action

- Dietary myoinositol and phytate may protect against fatty liver by inhibiting lipogenesis.[156] These forms of inositol suppressed rises in liver lipids and lipogenic enzymes in sucrose-fed rats, but did not prevent orotic acid-induced liver lipid accumulation suggesting they act to decrease lipid production in the liver rather than increase lipid secretion.

- In addition to decreasing cellular proliferation, IP6 also stimulates reversion of malignant mammalian cells to the normal phenotype, *in vitro*.[292] The anticancer action of phosphorylated forms of inositol probably involves numerous signal transduction pathways, cell cycle regulatory genes, differentiation genes, oncogenes, and possibly tumor suppressor genes.

22.4 Research

22.4.1 Inositol and Fatty Liver

High dietary sucrose is known to induce fatty liver in rats. Both free inositol and phytic acid have been shown to reduce liver lipids and decrease liver lipogenic enzyme activities in rats fed a high sucrose diet for 12-14 days.[156] Table 22.1 summarizes the results. The fact that both free inositol and phytic acid had similar effects on the parameters measured suggests that they act on lipid metabolism in a similar way. Interestingly, these effects were not observed for dietary cornstarch, a polymer of sucrose.

Inositol and phytate lower lipids by inhibiting lipogenesis rather than increasing lipid secretion. Orotic acid is an agent that causes liver lipid accumulation by severe inhibition of liver lipoprotein secretion without affecting lipogenesis. Yet, phytic acid and inositol do not prevent orotic acid-induced liver lipid accumulation in rats. Conversely, **DDT pesticide-induced lipid accumulation, which is a result of increased lipogenesis, is inhibited by these compounds.**[156]

Results by Jariwalla et al[140] support a lipid-lowering role for IP6 (phytate) in serum as well. Serum total cholesterol and triglycerides were lowered by 31.8% and 64.0%, respectively, in rats on a cholesterol-enriched diet when the diet was supplemented with 8.9% phytic acid by weight.

22.4.2 Inositol and Carcinogenesis

Nishino et al[239] reported that myoinositol supplied in drinking water significantly reduced lung and liver carcinogenesis in mice. For the examination of lung carcinogenesis, researchers administered 4-nitroquinoline 1-oxide (4NQO) to male ddY mice to initiate lung carcinogenesis, followed by promotion of tumorigenesis by daily administration of 10% glycerol in water for 25 weeks. During the promotion period, experimental mice were given myoinositol at a concentration of 1% in drinking water. To examine liver carcinogenesis, the researchers used male C3H/He mice that had a high incidence of spontaneous liver tumorigenesis. These mice were given 1% myoinositol in their drinking water for 40 weeks. Control mice in both experiments

Treatment	Liver total lipid (mg/g tissue)	Liver triglyceride (μmol/g tissue)	Liver G6PD (mU/mg protein)[2]	Liver FAS (mU/mg protein)[2]	Liver CBX (mU/mg protein)[2]
Sucrose alone	94.2[a]	61.4[a]	105.5[a]	6.11[a]	6.12[b]
Sucrose + myoinositol	47.4[b]	11.6[b]	64.2[b]	4.31[b]	4.91[b]
Sucrose + phytate	45.7[b]	10.4[b]	58.2[b]	3.78[b]	5.14[b]
Pooled SEM	5.3	5.3	6.6	0.54	0.51

G6PD=glucose-6-phosphate dehydrogenase; FAS=fatty acid synthetase; CBX=acetyl-CoA carboxylase.
Within a column, values followed by the same letter are not significantly different ($p<0.05$).
1 mU of enzyme is the amount of enzyme required to produce 1 nmol of measured product per minute at 25°C, except for CBX, which was measured at 37°C.

Table 22.1
*Effects of dietary addition of 5.6 mmol/kg myoinositol (0.1%) or phytate (0.37%)
on liver lipid levels and lipogenic enzyme activities. Adapted from Katayama et al.[156]*

received the same treatment as experimental mice but without myoinositol supplementation. At autopsy, the researchers counted the number of mice with tumors and the number of tumors per mouse. Myoinositol significantly lowered the number of tumors per mouse but not the incidence of tumor-bearing mice in the lung carcinogenesis experiment. However, myoinositol reduced both the number of tumor-bearing mice and the number of tumors per mouse in the spontaneous liver carcinogenesis experiment. Table 22.2 summarizes the data for both experiments.

Treatment	N	No. of Tumor-bearing mice (%)	Tumors per mouse
Induced lung carcinogenesis in ddY mice			
Control	12	11 (92)	4.9[a]
1% myoinositol	12	9 (75)	2.0[a]
Spontaneous liver carcinogenesis in C3H/He mice			
Control	17	15 (88)[a]	7.8[b]
1% myoinositol	13	5 (38)[a]	0.8[b]
[a] (p<0.05) [b] (p<0.01)			

Table 22.2
Effect of myoinositol on chemically-induced lung carcinogenesis and spontaneous liver carcinogenesis in mice. Adapted from Nishino, H et al.[239]

22.5 Overview

These clinical results coupled with the results of earlier trials strongly suggest that **inositol:**

- Protects against fatty liver
- Prevents liver carcinogenesis

22.5.1 Contraindications

- None known

22.5.2 Side effects

• None known

22.5.3 Possible Interactions with Drugs

• None known

22.5.4 Possible Interactions with Herbs and other Dietary Supplements

• Insufficient reliable information

22.5.6 Possible Interactions with Foods

• Phytic acid, the form of inositol found in many foods, may interfere with absorption of minerals, especially calcium, zinc, and iron.[141]

22.5.7 Possible Interactions with Diseases or Conditions

• None known

22.5.8 Typical Dosage

• 12-18 g per day have been used in the treatment of disorders related to inositol metabolism.[141]

PART 2
CLINICAL REFERENCES

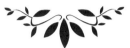

(CHAPTERS 6-22)

1. Abdel-Salam, O. M. et al. 1999. Capsaicin-sensitive afferent sensory nerves in modulating gastric mucosal defense against noxious agents. *J Physiol Paris* 93(5): 443-454.
2. Adlercreutz, H. et al. 1982. Excretion of the lignans enterolactone and enterodiol and of equol in omnivorous and vegetarian postmenopausal women and in women with breast cancer. *Lancet* 2(8311): 1295-1299.
3. Adlercreutz, H. et al. 1986. Determination of urinary lignans and phytoestrogen metabolites, potential antiestrogens and anticarcinogens, in urine of women on various habitual diets. *J Steroid Biochem* 25(5B): 791-797.
4. Adlercreutz, H. et al. 1987. Effect of dietary components, including lignans and phytoestrogens, on enterohepatic circulation and liver metabolism of estrogens and on sex hormone binding globulin (SHBG). *J Steroid Biochem* 27(4-6): 1135-1144.
5. Adlercreutz, H. et al. 1988. Association between dietary fiber, urinary excretion of lignans and isoflavonic phytoestrogens, and plasma non-protein bound sex hormones in relation to breast cancer. In: Bresciani, F. et al. (Eds.). Progress in Cancer Research and Therapy: Hormones and Cancer 3, vol. 35. New York: Raven Press. 409-412.
6. Adlercreutz, H. et al. 1992. Dietary phytoestrogens and cancer: In vitro and in vivo studies. *J Steroid Biochem Mol Biol* 41(3-8): 331-337.
7. Adlercreutz, H. et al. 1993. Inhibition of human aromatase by mammalian lignans and isoflavonoid phytoestrogens. *J Steroid Biochem Mol Biol* 44(2): 147-153.
8. Adlercreutz, C. H. et al. 1995a. Soybean phytoestrogen intake and cancer risk. *J Nutr* 125(3 Suppl): 757S-770S.
9. Adlercreutz, H. 1995b. Phytoestrogens: Epidemiology and a possible role in cancer protection. *Environ Health Perspect* 103 Suppl.
10. Adlercreutz, H. et al. 1995c. Isotope dilution gas chromatographic-mass spectrometric method for the determination of unconjugated lignans and isoflavonoids in human feces, with preliminary results in omnivorous and vegetarian women. *Anal Biochem* 225(1): 101-108.
11. Ahmad, N. et al. 1998. Skin cancer chemopreventive effects of a flavonoid antioxidant silymarin are mediated via impairment of receptor tyrosine kinase signaling and perturbation in cell cycle progression. *Biochem Biophys Res Commun* 247(2): 294-301.
12. Alcorn, J. B. 1984. Huastec Mayan Ethnobotany. Austin, TX: University of Texas Press. 578-580.
13. Allen, S. D. and E. J. Baron. 1991. *Clostridium*. In: Balows, A. et al. (Eds.), Manual of Clinical Microbiology. 5th ed. Washington, DC: American Society for Microbiology. 505-521.
14. Alonso-Aperte, E. and G. Varela-Moreiras. 1996. Brain folates and DNA methylation in rats fed a choline deficient diet or treated with low doses of methotrexate. *Int J Vitam Nutr Res* 66(3): 232-236.
15. Alving, K. et al. 1991. Capsaicin-induced local effector responses, autonomic reflexes and sensory neuropeptide depletion in the pig. *Naunyn Schmiedebergs Arch Pharmacol* 343(1): 37-45.
16. Amara-Mokrane, Y. A. et al. 1996. Protective effects of alpha-hederin, chlorophyllin, and ascorbic acid towards the induction of micronuclei by doxorubicin in cultured human lymphocytes. *Mutagenesis* 11(2): 161-167.
17. Anderson, D. M. et al. (eds.). 2000a. Dorland's Illustrated Medical Dictionary, 26th ed. Philadelphia: W. B. Saunders, Co.
18. Anderson, J. W. 1987. Dietary fiber, lipids, and atherosclerosis. *Am J Cardiol* 60(12): 17G-22G.
19. Anderson, J. W. et al. 1992. Cholesterol-lowering effects of psyllium-enriched cereal as an adjunct to a prudent diet in the treatment of mild to moderate hypercholesterolemia. *Am J Clin Nutr* 56(1): 93-98.
20. Anderson, J. W. 1995a. Dietary fibre, complex carbohydrate and coronary artery disease. *Can J Cardiol* 11 Suppl G: 55G-62G.
21. Anderson, J. W. 1995b. Short-chain fatty acids and lipid metabolism. In: Cummings, J. H. et al., eds. Physiological and clinical aspects of short-chain fatty acids. New York: Cambridge University Press. 509-523.
22. Anderson, J. W. et al. 2000b. Cholesterol-lowering effects of psyllium intake adjunctive to diet therapy in men and women with hypercholesterolemia: Meta-analysis of 8 controlled trials. *Am J Clin Nutr* 71(2): 472-479.
23. Aritsuka, T. et al., 1989. Effect of beet dietary fiber on lipid metabolism in rats fed a cholesterol-free diet in comparison with pectin and cellulose. *J Jpn Soc Nutr Food Sci* 42(4): 295-304.
24. Asai, A. et al. 1999. Antioxidative effects of turmeric, rosemary, and capsicum extracts on membrane phospholipid peroxidation and liver lipid metabolism in mice. *Biosci Biotechnol Biochem* 63(12): 2118-2122.
25. Barnes, S. et al. 1990. Soybeans inhibit mammary tumors in models of breast cancer. *Prog Clin Biol Res* 347: 239-253.

26. Beecher, C. W. W. 1994. Cancer preventive properties of varieties of Brassica oleracea: A review. *Am J Clin Nutr* 59(5S): 1166S-1170S.

27. Benninger, J. et al. 1999. Acute hepatitis induced by Greater Celandine (*Chelidonium majus*). *Gastroenterology* 117(5): 1234-1237.

28. Bernstein, J. E. et al. 1987. Treatment of chronic postherpetic neuralgia with topical capsaicin. A preliminary study. *J Am Acad Dermatol* 17(1): 93-96.

29. Block, G. et al. 1992. Fruit, vegetables, and cancer prevention: A review of the epidemiological evidence. *Nutr Cancer* 18(1): 1-29.

30. Blumenthal, M. et al. (Eds.). 2000. Herbal Medicine: Expanded Commission E Monographs. Austin, TX: American Botanical Council.

31. Bobek, P. et al. 2000. The effect of red beet (Beta vulgaris var. rubra) fiber on alimentary hypercholesterolemia and chemically induced colon carcinogenesis in rats. Nahrung, 44(3): 184-187.

32. Bouraoui, A. et al. 1988. Effects of capsicum fruit on theophylline absorption and bioavailability in rabbits. *Drug Nutr Interact* 5(4): 345-350.

33. Bourne, N. et al. 1999. Civamide (cis-capsaicin) for treatment of primary or recurrent experimental genital herpes. *Antimicrob Agents Chemother* 43(11): 2685-2688.

34. Broca, C. et al. 1999. 4-hydroxyisoleucine: Experimental evidence of its insulinotropic and antidiabetic properties. *Am J Physiol* 277(4 Pt 1): E617-E623.

35. Broca, C. et al. 2000. 4-hydroxyisoleucine: Effects of synthetic and natural analogues on insulin secretion. *Eur J Pharmacol* 390(3): 339-345.

36. Brown, R. 1997. Potential interactions of herbal medicines with antipsychotics, antidepressants, and hypnotics. *Euro J Herbal Med* 3:25-28.

37. Buchman, A. L. et al. 1995. Choline deficiency: A cause of hepatic steatosis during parenteral nutrition that can be reversed with intravenous choline supplementation. *Hepatology* 22(5): 1399-1403.

38. Buckley, A. R. et al. 1993. Inhibition by genistein of prolactin-induced Nb2 lymphoma cell mitogenesis. *Mol Cell Endocrinol* 98(1): 17-25.

39. Buddington, R. K. et al. 1999. Influence of fermentable fiber on small intestinal dimensions and transport of glucose and proline in dogs. *Am J Vet Res* 60(3): 354-358.

40. Budzinski, J. W. et al. 2000. An in vitro evaluation of human cytochrome P450 3A4 inhibition by selected commercial herbal extracts and tinctures. Phytomedicine 7(4): 273-282.

41. Buhman, K. K. et al. 1998. Dietary psyllium increases fecal bile acid excretion, total steroid excretion, and bile acid biosynthesis in rats. *J Nutr* 128(7): 1199-1203.

42. But, P. P. H. et al. (Eds.). 1997. International Collation of Traditional and Folk Medicine. Singapore: World Scientific. 138-139.

43. Butland, B. K. et al. 2000. Diet, lung function, and lung function decline in a cohort of 2512 middle aged men. *Thorax* 55(2): 102-108.

44. Cadenas, S. et al. 1994. Caloric and carbohydrate restriction in the kidney: Effects on free radical metabolism. *Exp Gerontol* 29(1): 77-88.

45. Campbell, D. R. and M. S. Kurzer. 1993. Flavonoid inhibition of aromatase enzyme activity in human preadipocytes. *J Steroid Biochem Mol Biol* 46(3): 381-388.

46. Canty, D. J. and S. H. Zeisel. 1994. Lecithin and choline in human health and disease. *Nutr Rev* 52(10): 327-339.

47. Casanova, M. et al. 1999. Developmental effects of dietary phytoestrogens in Sprague-Dawley rats and interactions of genistein and daidzein with rat estrogen receptors alpha and beta in vitro. *Toxicol Sci* 51(2): 236-244.

48. Cassady, J. M. et al. 1988. Use of a mammalian cell culture benzo(a)pyrene metabolism assay for the detection of potential anticarcinogens from natural products: Inhibition of metabolism by biochanin A, an isoflavone from Trifolium pratense L. *Cancer Res* 48(22): 6257-6261.

49. Cerutti, P. A. 1994. Oxy-radicals and cancer. *Lancet* 344(8926): 862-863.

50. Chae, Y. H. et al. 1991. Effects of biochanin A on metabolism, DNA binding and mutagenicity of benzo[a]pyrene in mammalian cell cultures. *Carcinogenesis* 12(11): 2001-2006.

51. Chandar, N. and B. Lombardi. 1988. Liver cell proliferation and incidence of hepatocellular carcinomas in rats fed consecutively a choline-devoid and a choline-supplemented diet. *Carcinogenesis* 9(2): 259-263.

52. Chandar, N. et al. 1989. c-myc gene amplification during hepatocarcinogenesis by a choline-devoid diet. *Proc Natl Acad Sci USA* 86(8): 2703-2707.

53. Chen, W-J. L. et al. 1984. Propionate may mediate the hypocholesterolemic effects of certain soluble plant fibers in cholesterol-fed rats. *Proc Soc Exp Biol Med* 175(2): 215-218.

54. Cherbut, C. et al. 1994. Involvement of small intestinal motility in blood glucose response to dietary fibre in man. *Br J Nutr* 71(5): 675-685.

55. Christensen, B. et al. 1999. Whole blood folate, homocysteine in serum, and risk of first acute myocardial infarction. *Atherosclerosis* 147(2): 317-326

56. Chung, W. et al. 2000. Protective effects of hemin and tetrakis(4-benzoic acid)porphyrin on bacterial mutagenesis and mouse skin carcinogenesis induced by 7,12-dimethylbenz[a]anthracene. *Mutat Res* 472(1-2): 139-145.

57. Chyou, P. H. et al. 1990. A case-cohort study of diet and stomach cancer. *Cancer Res* 50(23): 7501-7504.

58. Cichewicz, R. H. and P. A. Thorpe. 1996. The antimicrobial properties of chile peppers (Capsicum species) and their uses in Mayan medicine. *J Ethnopharmacol* 52(2): 61-70.

59. Colditz, G. A. et al. 1985. Increased green and yellow vegetable intake and lowered cancer deaths in an elderly population. *Am J Clin Nutr* 41(1): 32-36.

60. Constantinou, A. et al. 1990. Induction of differentiation and DNA strand breakage in human HL-60 and K-562 leukemia cells by genistein. *Cancer Res* 50(9): 2618-2624.

61. Cordell, G. A. and O. E. Araujo. 1993. Capsaicin: Identification, nomenclature, and pharmacotherapy. *Ann Pharmacother* 27(3): 330-336.

62. Cruz, L. et al. 1999. Ingestion of chilli pepper (Capsicum annuum) reduces salicylate bioavailability after oral aspirin administration in the rat. *Can J Physiol Pharmacol* 77(6): 441-446.

63. Dashwood, R. and C. Liew. 1992. Chlorophyllin-enhanced excretion of urinary and fecal mutagens in rats given 2-amino-3-methylimidazo[4,5]quinoline. *Environ Mol Mutagen* 20(3): 199-205.

64. Dashwood, R. H. 1998. Indole-3-carbinol: Anticarcinogen or tumor promoter in brassica vegetables? *Chem Biol Interact* 110(1-2): 1-5.

65. Day, G. L. et al. 1994. Dietary factors and second primary cancers: a follow-up of oral and pharyngeal cancer patients. *Nutr Cancer* 21(3): 223-232.

66. De, A. K. and J. J. Ghosh. 1989. Capsaicin pretreatment protects free radical induced rat lung damage on exposure to gaseous chemical lung irritants. *Phytother Res* 3: 159-161.

67. De, A. K. and J. J. Ghosh. 1992. Studies on capsaicin inhibition of chemically induced lipid peroxidation in the lung and liver tissues of rat. *Phytother Res* 6: 34-37.

68. De, A. K. et al. 1995. Inhibition by capsaicin against cyclophosphamide-induced clastogenicity and DNA damage in mice. *Mutat Res* 335(3): 253-258.

69. Debreceni, A. et al. 1999. Capsaicin increases gastric emptying rate in healthy human subjects measured by 13C-labeled octanoic acid breath test. *J Physiol Paris* 93(5): 455-460.

70. Der Marderosian, A. (ed.). 1999. The Review of Natural Products. St. Louis: Facts and Comparisons.

71. Dixon-Shanies, D. and N. Shaikh. 1999. Growth inhibition of human breast cancer cells by herbs and phytoestrogens. *Oncol Rep* 6(6): 1383-1387.

72. Doucet, E. and A. Tremblay. 1997. Food intake, energy balance and body weight control. *Eur J Clin Nutr* 51(12): 846-855.

73. Draper, C. et al. 1997. Phytoestrogens reduce bone loss and bone resorption in oophorectomized rats. *J Nutr* 127(9): 1795-1799.

74. Dubey, R. K. et al. 1998. 17 b-estradiol, its metabolites, and progesterone inhibit cardiac fibroblast growth. *Hypertension* 31(1 Pt 2): 522-528.

75. Dubey, R. K. et al. 1999. Phytoestrogens inhibit growth and MAP kinase activity in human aortic smooth muscle cells. *Hypertension* 33(1 Pt 2): 177-182.

76. Duke, J. 2000. Dr. Duke's Phytochemical and Ethnobotanical Databases. Beltsville, Maryland: USDA-ARS-NGRL-Beltsville Agricultural Research Service.

77. Ellingwood, F. 1898. A Systematic Treatise on Materia Medica and Therapeutics With Reference to the Most Direct Action of Drugs. Chicago: Chicago Medical Press Co.

78. Ellingwood, F. 1919. New American Materia Medica Therapeutics and Pharmacognosy. Chicago: Ellingwood's Therapeutist.

79. Ely, H. 1989. Dermatologic therapies you've probably never heard of. *Dermatol Clin* 7(1): 19-35.

80. Emerit, I. and P. A. Cerutti. 1982. Tumor promoter phorbol 12-myristate 13-acetate induces a clastogenic factor in human lymphocytes. *Proc Natl Acad Sci USA* 79(23): 7509-7513.

81. Esaki, H. and H. Onozaki. 1982. Antimicrobial action of pungent principles in radish root (Raphanus sativus). *J Jpn Soc Food Nutr* 35(3): 207-211.

82. ESCOP. 1997. Juniperi fructus. Monographs on the Medicinal Uses of Plant Drugs. Exter, UK: European Scientific Cooperative on Phytotherapy.

83. Espinosa-Aguirre, J. J. et al. 1993. Mutagenic activity of urban air samples and its modulation by chili extracts. *Mutat Res* 303(2): 55-61.

84. Everson, G. T. et al. 1992. Effects of psyllium hydrophilic mucilloid on LDL-cholesterol and bile acid synthesis in hypercholesterolemic men. *J Lipid Res* 33(8): 1183-1192.

85. Fahey, J. W. et al. 1997. Broccoli sprouts: An exceptionally rich source of inducers of enzymes that protect against chemical carcinogens. *Proc Natl Acad Sci USA* 94(19): 10367-10372.

86. Fernandez-Banares, F. et al. 1999. Randomized clinical trial of Plantago ovata seeds (dietary fiber) as compared with mesalamine in maintaining remission in ulcerative colitis. *Am J Gastroenterol* 94(2): 427-433.

87. Figtree, G. A. et al. 2000. Plant-derived estrogens relax coronary arteries in vitro by a calcium antagonistic mechanism. *J Am Coll Cardiol* 35(7): 1977-1985.

88. Fleming, T. (Ed.). 2000. PDR for Herbal Medicines, 2nd ed. Montvale, NJ: Medical Economics Company. 656-657.

89. Foldeak, S. and G. Dombradi. 1964. Tumor-growth inhibiting substances of plant origin. Isolation of the active principle of Arctium lappa. *Acta Phys Chem* 10: 91-93.

90. Foster, S. 1996. Milk thistle, Silybum marianum, Botanical Series No. 305. Austin, TX: American Botanical Council.

91. Fotsis, T. et al. 1993. Genistein, a dietary-derived inhibitor of in vitro angiogenesis. *Proc Natl Acad Sci USA* 90(7): 2690-2694.

92. Francis, A. R. et al. 1989a. Modifying role of dietary factors on the mutagenicity of aflatoxin B1: in vitro effect of plant flavonoids. *Mutat Res* 222(4): 393-401.

93. Francis, A. R. et al. 1989b. Modulating effect of plant flavonoids on the mutagenicity of N-methyl-N'-nitro-N-nitrosoguanidine. *Carcinogenesis* 10(10): 1953-1955.

94. Frankel, S. et al. 1998. Childhood energy intake and adult mortality from cancer: The Boyd Orr Cohort Study. *BMJ* 316(7130): 499-504.

95. Fuhr, U. 1998. Drug interactions with grapefruit juice. Extent, probable mechanism and clinical relevance. *Drug Saf* 18(4):251-272.

96. Fukushima, M. et al. 2000. Hepatic LDL receptor mRNA in rats is increased by dietary mushroom (Agaricus bisporus) fiber and sugar beet fiber. *J Nutr* 130(9): 2151-2156.

97. Fung, M. C. et al. 1997. Effects of biochanin A on the growth and differentiation of myeloid leukemia WEHI-3B (JCS) cells. *Life Sci* 61(2): 105-115.

98. Ganji, V. and C. V. Kies. 1994. Psyllium husk fiber supplementation to soybean and coconut oil diets of humans: Effect on fat digestibility and faecal fatty acid excretion. *Eur J Clin Nutr* 48(8): 595-597.

99. Ganji, V. and C. V. Kies. 1996. Psyllium husk fiber supplementation to the diets rich in soybean or coconut oil: Hypocholesterolemic effect in healthy humans. *Int J Food Sci Nutr* 47(2): 103-110.

100. Gardner, D. R. et al. 1998. Abortifacient effects of lodgepole pine (Pinus contorta) and common juniper (Juniperus communis) on cattle. *Vet Hum Toxicol* 40(5): 260-263.

101. Ghoshal, A. K. and E. Farber. 1984. The induction of liver cancer by dietary deficiency of choline and methionine without added carcinogens. *Carcinogenesis* 5(10): 1367-1370.

102. Ghoshal A. K. et al. 1990. Prevention by free radical scavenger AD5 of prooxidant effects of choline deficiency. *Free Radic Biol Med* 8(1): 3-7.

103. Ghoshal, A. K. 1995. New insight into the biochemical pathology of liver in choline deficiency. *Crit Rev Biochem Mol Biol* 30(4): 263-273.

104. Giles, D. and H. Wei. 1997. Effect of structurally related flavones/isoflavones on hydrogen peroxide production and oxidative DNA damage in phorbol ester-stimulated HL-60 cells. *Nutr Cancer* 29(1): 77-82.

105. Gilmore, M. R. 1919. Uses of plants by the Indians of the Missouri River region. SI-BAE Annual Report #33.

106. Glore, S. R. et al. 1994. Soluble fiber and serum lipids: A literature review. *J Am Diet Assoc* 94(4): 425-436.

107. Gong, X. et al. 1997. Antioxidant enzyme activities in lens, liver, and kidney of caloric restricted Emory mice. *Mech Ageing Dev* 99(3): 181-192.

108. Gopalan, R. et al. 1991. Serum lipid and lipoprotein fractions in bengal gram and biochanin A induced alterations in atherosclerosis. *Indian Heart J* 43(3): 185-189.

109. Grases, F. et al. 1994. Urolithiasis and phytotherapy. *Int Urol Nephrol* 26(5): 507-511.

110. Grattagliano, I. et al. 2000. Starvation impairs antioxidnt defense in fatty livers of rats fed a choline-deficient diet. *J Nutr* 130(9): 2131-2136.

111. Grubbs, C. J. 1995. Chemoprevention of chemically induced mammary cancinogenesis by indole-3-carbinol. *Anticancer Res* 15(3): 709-716.

112. Gruenwald, J. et al. 1998. PDR for Herbal Medicines, 1st ed. Montvale, NJ: Medical Economics Company, Inc.

113. Gupta, D. et al. 1999. Modulation of some gluconeogenic enzyme activities in diabetic rat liver and kidney: Effects of antidiabetic compounds. *Indian J Exp Biol* 37(2): 196-199.

114. Hagiwara, Y. 1985. In Passwater, R. A. (Ed.). A good health guide. New Canaan, CT: Keats Publishing, Inc.

115. Halliwell, B. and J. M. C. Gutteridge. 1984. Lipid peroxidation, oxygen radicals, cell damage and antioxidant therapy. *Lancet* 1: 1396-1397.

116. Harman, D. 1981. The aging process. *Proc Natl Acad Sci USA* 78(11): 7124-7128.

117. Hart, R. W. and A. Turturro. 1997. Dietary restrictions and cancer. *Environ Health Perspect* 105 Suppl 4: 989-992.

118. Hawrylewicz, E. J. et al. 1991. Dietary soybean isolate and methionine supplementation affect mammary tumor progression in rats. *J Nutr* 121(10): 1693-1698.

119. Hayatsu, H. et al. 1993. Porphyrins as potential inhibitors against exposure to carcinogens and mutagens. *Mutat Res* 290(1): 79-85.

120. He, K. et al. 1998. Inactivation of cytochrome P450 3A4 by bergamottin, a component of grapefruit juice. *Chem Res Toxicol* 11(4): 252-259.

121. Heck, A. M. et al.. 2000. Potential interactions between alternative therapies and warfarin. *Am J Health Syst Pharm* 57(13): 1221-1227.

122. Hempstock, J. et al. 1998. Growth inhibition of prostate cell lines in vitro by phytooestrogens. *Br J Urol* 82(4): 560-563.

123. Hensel, A. and K. Meier. 1999. Pectins and xyloglucans exhibit antimutagenic activities against nitroaromatic compounds. *Planta Med* 65(5): 395-399.

124. Hiller, K. O. et al. 1998. Antispasmodic and relaxant activity of chelidonine, protopine, coptisine, and Chelidonium majus extracts on isolated guinea-pig ileum. *Planta Med* 64(8): 758-760.

125. Hirano, T. et al. 1989a. Effects of synthetic and naturally occurring flavonoids on mitogen-induced proliferation of human peripheral-blood lymphocytes. *Life Sci* 45(15): 1407-1411.

126. Hirano, T. et al. 1989b. Antiproliferative effects of synthetic and naturally occurring flavonoids on tumor cells of the human breast carcinoma cell line, ZR-75-1. *Res Commun Chem Pathol Pharmacol* 64(1): 69-78.

127. Hirano, T. et al. 1991. Suppression of mitogen-induced proliferation of human peripheral blood lymphocytes by plant lignans. *Planta Med* 57(4): 331-334.

128. Hirose, M. et al. 2000. Effects of arctiin on PhIP-induced mammary, colon and pancreatic carcinogenesis in female Sprague-Dawley rats and MeIQx-induced hepatocarcinogenesis in male F344 rats. *Cancer Lett* 155(1): 79-88.

129. Holub, B. J. 1982. The nutritional significance, metabolism, and function of myo-inositol and phosphatidylinositol in health and disease. *Adv Nutr Res* 4: 107-141.

130. Honma, Y. et al. 1990. Inhibition of abl oncogene tyrosine kinase induces erythroid differentiation of human myelogenous leukemia K562 cells. *Jpn J Cancer Res* 81: 1132-1136.

131. Horowitz, M. et al. 1992. The effect of chilli on gastrointestinal transit. *J Gastroenterol Hepatol* 7(1): 52-56.

132. Hsieh, L. L. et al. 1989. Altered expression of retrovirus-like sequences and cellular oncogenes in mice fed methyl-deficient diets. *Cancer Res* 49(14): 3795-3799.

133. Hsu, J. T. et al. 2000. Regulation of inducible nitric oxide synthase by dietary phytoestrogen in MCF-7 human mammary cancer cells. *Reprod Nutr Dev* 40(1): 11-18.

134. Hur, H. and F. Rafii. 2000. Biotransformation of the isoflavonoids biochanin A, formononetin, and glycitein by eubacterium limosum. *FEMS Microbiol Lett* 192(1): 21-25.

135. Hussain, M. S. and N. Chandrasekhara. 1994. Biliary proteins from hepatic bile of rats fed curcumin or capsaicin inhibit cholesterol crystal nucleation in supersaturated model bile. *Indian J Biochem Biophys* 31(5): 407-412.

136. Iwahashi, H. et al. 1990. Effects of caffeic acid and its related catechols on OH· formation by 3-hydroxy-anthranilic acid, FeCl3 and hydrogen peroxide. *Arch Biochem Biophys* 276: 242-247.

137. Iwakami, S. et al. 1992. Platelet activating factor (PAF) antagonists contained in medicinal plants: Lignans and sesquiterpenes. *Chem Pharm Bull* (Tokyo) 40(5): 1196-1198.

138. Iwu, M.M. 1990. Handbook of African Medicinal Plants. Boca Raton: CRC Press. 139–140.

139. Jang, J. J. et al. 1989. Inhibitory effect of capsaicin on mouse lung tumor development. *In Vivo* 3(1): 49-53.

140. Jariwalla, R. J. 1999. Inositol hexaphosphate (IP6) as an antineoplastic and lipid-lowering agent. *Anti Br J Nutr* 19: 3699-3702.

141. Jellin, J. M. et al. 2000. Pharmacist's Letter/Prescriber's Letter Natural Medicines Comprehensive Database. 3rd ed. Stockton, CA: Therapeutic Research Faculty. 223-225.

142. Jensen-Jarolim, E. et al. 1998. Bell peppers (Capsicum annuum) express allergens (profilin, pathogenesis-related protein P23 and Bet v 1) depending on the horticultural strain. *Int Arch Allergy Immunol* 116(2): 103-109.

143. Jing, Y. et al. 1993. Differentiation of promyelocytic leukemia cells HL-60 induced by daidzein in vitro and in vivo. *Anticancer Res* 13(4): 1049-1054.

144. Jones, S. M. et al. 1998. Dietary juniper berry oil minimizes hepatic reperfusion injury in the rat. *Hepatology* 28(4): 1042-1050.

145. Kagan, V. E. et al. 1990. Recycling and anti-oxidant activity of tocopherol homologs of differing hydrocarbon chain lengths in liver microsomes. *Arch Biochem Biophys* 282: 221-225.

146. Kallela, K. et al. 1984. Plant oestrogens; the cause of decreased fertility in cows. A case report. *Nord Vet Med* 36(3-4): 124-129.

147. Kameoka, S. et al. 1999. Expression of antioxidant proteins in human intestinal Caco-2 cells treated with dietary flavonoids. *Cancer Lett* 146(2): 161-167.

148. Kanatani, Y. et al. 1993. Genistein exhibits preferential cytotoxicity to a leukemogenic variant but induces differentiation of a non-leukemogenic variant of the mouse monocytic leukemia Mm cell line. *Leuk Res* 17(10): 847-853.

149. Kanauchi, O. et al. 2001. Germinated barley foodstuff feeding. A novel neutraceutical therapeutic strategy for ulcerative colitis. *Digestion* 63(Suppl): 60-67.

150. Kang, J. Y. et al. 1995a. Effect of capsaicin and chilli on ethanol induced gastric mucosal injury in the rat. *Gut* 36(5): 664-669.

151. Kang, J. Y. et al. 1995b. Chili—protective factor against peptic ulcer? *Dig Dis Sci* 40(3): 576-579.

152. Kang, J. Y. et al. 1996. Effect of capsaicin and cimetidine on the healing of acetic acid induced gastric ulceration in the rat. *Gut* 38(6): 832-836.

153. Kapoor, L. D. 1990. Handbook of Ayurvedic Medicinal Plants. Boca Raton: CRC Press. 98.

154. Karnick, C. R. 1994. Pharmacopoeial Standards of Herbal Plants, Vol. 1. Delhi: Sri Satguru Publications. 79-80.

155. Kasai, H.et al. 2000. Action of chlorogenic acid in vegetables and fruits as an inhibitor of 8-hydroxydeoxyguanosine formation in vitro and in a rat carcinogenesis model. *Food Chem Toxicol* 38(5): 467-471.

156. Katayama, T. 1999. Hypolipidemic action of phytic acid (IP6): Prevention of fatty liver. *Anticancer Res* 19(5A): 3695-3698.

157. Katiyar, S. K. et al. 1997. Protective effects of silymarin against photocarcinogenesis in a mouse skin model. *J Natl Cancer Inst* 89(8): 556-566.

158. Kawada, T. et al. 1988. Some pungent principles of spices cause the adrenal medulla to secrete catecholamine in anesthetized rats. *Proc Soc Exp Biol Med* 188(2): 229-233.

159. Kensler, T. W. and B. G. Taffe. 1989. Role of free radicals in tumor promotion and progression. *Prog Clin Biol Res* 298: 233-248.

160. Khan, K. I. et al. 1985. The antimicrobial activity of allium-sativum garlic, allium-cepa onion, and raphanus-sativus radish. *J Pharm* (Lahore) 6(1-2): 59-72.

161. Kiguchi, K. et al. 1990. Genistein-induced cell differentiation and protein-linked DNA strand breakage in human melanoma cells. *Cancer Commun* 2(8): 271-277.

162. Kim, J. D. et al. 1996. Exercise and diet modulate cardiac lipid peroxidation and antioxidant defenses. *Free Radic Biol Med* 20(1): 83-88.

163. Klopfenstein, C. F. 1990. Nutritional properties of coarse and fine sugar beet fiber and hard red wheat bran. I. Effects on rat serum and liver cholesterol and triglycerides and on fecal characteristics. *Cereal Chem* 67(6): 538-541.

164. Kochhar, K. P. et al. 1999. Gastro-intestinal effects of Indian spice mixture (Garam Masala). *Trop Gastroenterol* 20(4): 170-174.

165. Kondo, K. et al. 1991. Induction of in vitro differentiation of mouse embryonal carcinoma (F9) cells by inhibitors of topoisomerases. *Cancer Res* 51(19): 5398-5404.

166. Krecman, V. et al. 1998. Silymarin inhibits the development of diet-induced hypercholesterolemia in rats. *Planta Med* 64(2): 138-142.

167. Kritchevsky, D. et al. 1995. Influence of psyllium preparations on plasma and liver lipids of cholesterol-fed rats. *Artery* 21(6): 303-311.

168. Kuiper, G. G. et al. 1998. Interaction of estrogenic chemicals and phytoestrogens with estrogen receptor beta. *Endocrinology* 139(10): 4252-4263.

169. Kuriu, A. et al. 1991. Proliferation of human myeloid leukemia cell line associated with the tyrosine-phosphorylation and activation of the proto-oncogene c-kit product. *Blood* 78(11): 2834-2840.

170. Kurzer, M. S. and X. Xu. 1997. Dietary phytoestrogens. *Annu Rev Nutr* 17: 353-381.

171. Kusano, T. et al. 1974. Nutritive components of buckwheat. *J Jap Soc Food Nutr* 27(9): 461-465.

172. Kvåle, G. et al. 1983. Dietary habits and lung cancer risk. *Int J Cancer* 31(4): 397-405.

173. La, M. and M. J. Rand. 1993. Neurogenic vasodilation in isolated perfused segments of rabbit jejunal artery. *Clin Exp Pharmacol Physiol* 20(5): 355-358.

174. Laganiere, S. and B. P. Yu. 1989. Effect of chronic food restriction in aging rats. II. Liver cytosolic antioxidants and related enzymes. *Mech Ageing Dev* 48(3): 221-230.

175. Lahiri-Chatterjee, M. et al. 1999. A flavonoid antioxidant, silymarin, affords exceptionally high protection against tumor promotion in the SENCAR mouse skin tumorigenesis model. *Cancer Res* 59(3): 622-632.

176. Landgren, F. et al. 1995. Plasma homocysteine in acute myocardial infarction: Homocysteine-lowering effect of folic acid. *J Intern Med* 237(4): 381-388.

177. Lang, I. et al. 1990. Immunomodulatory and hepatoprotective effects of in vivo treatment with free radical scavengers. *Ital J Gastroenterol* 22(5): 283-287.

178. Le Marchand, L. et al. 2000. Intake of flavonoids and lung cancer. *J Natl Cancer Inst* 92(2): 154-160.

179. Lee, H. P. et al. 1991. Dietary effects on breast-cancer risk in Singapore. *Lancet* 337(8751): 1197-1200.

180. Lee, D. W. and B. P. Yu. 1990. Modulation of free radicals and superoxide dismutases by age and dietary restriction. *Aging* (Milano) 2(4): 357-362.

181. Lee, M. and B. G. Devi. 1996. Effects of dietary restriction on experimental gastric mucosal injury in Fischer 344 rats. *Mech Ageing Dev* 89(1): 11-20.

182. Leitner, A. et al. 1998. Allergens in pepper and paprika: Immunologic investigation of the celery-birch-mugwort-spice syndrome. *Allergy* 53(1): 36-41.

183. Lembeck, F. 1987. Columbus, Capsicum and Capsaicin: Past, Present and Future. *Acta Physiol Hung* 69(3-4): 265-273.

184. Leng-Peschlow, E. 1996. Properties and medicinal use of flavonolignans (silymarin) from Silybum marianum. *Phytother Res* 10(Suppl): S25-S26.

185. Leontowicz, M. et al. 2001. Sugar beet pulp and apple pomace dietary fibers improve lipid metabolism in rats fed cholesterol. *Food Chemistry* 72(1): 73-78.

186. Leung, A.Y. and S. Foster. 1996. Encyclopedia of Common Natural Ingredients Used in Food, Drugs and Cosmetics, 2nd ed. New York: John Wiley & Sons, Inc.

187. Lim, K. et al. 1997. Dietary red pepper ingestion increases carbohydrate oxidation at rest and during exercise in runners. *Med Sci Sports Exerc* 29(3): 355-361.

188. Limlomwongse, L. et al. 1979. Effect of capsaicin on gastric acid secretion and mucosal blood flow in the rat. *J Nutr* 109(5): 773-777.

189. Lin, C. C. et al. 1996. Anti-inflammatory and radical scavenge effects of Arctium lappa. *Am J Chin Med* 24(2): 127-137.

190. Lin, H. J. et al. 1998. Glutathione transferase null genotype, broccoli, and lower prevalence of colorectal adenomas. *Cancer Epidemiol Biomarkers Prev* 7(8): 647-652.

191. Lin, S. C. et al. 2000. Hepatoprotective effects of Arctium lappa on carbon tetrachloride- and acetaminophen-induced liver damage. *Am J Chin Med* 28(2): 163-173.

192. Lorenz, D. et al. 1984. Pharmacokinetic studies with silymarin in human serum and bile. Methods Find Exp Clin Pharmacol 6(10): 655-661.

193. Lown, K. S. et al. 1997. Grapefruit juice increases felodipine oral availability in humans by decreasing intestinal CYP3A protein expression. *J Clin Invest* 99(10): 2545-2553.

194. Lugasi, A. 1998. Antioxidant and free radical scavenging properties of squeezed juice from black radish (Raphanus sativus L.) var niger) root. *Phytother Res* 12(7): 502-506.

195. Lynn, B. 1990. Capsaicin: Actions on nociceptive C-fibres and therapeutic potential. *Pain* 41(1): 61-69.

196. Ma, J. et al. 1997. Methylenetetrahydrofolate reductase polymorphism, dietary interactions, and risk of colorectal cancer. *Br J Nutr* 57(6): 1098-1102.

197. Mäkelä, S. et al. 1991. Role of plant estrogens in normal and estrogen-related altered growth of the mouse prostate. In: EURO FOOD TOX III. Proceedings of the Interdisciplinary Conference on Effects of Food on the Immune and Hormonal Systems. Institute of Toxicology, Swiss Federal Institute of Technology & University of Zürich, Schwerzenbach, Switzerland. 135-139.

198. Makishima, M. et al. 1991. Effects of inhibitors of protein tyrosine kinase activity and/or phosphatidylinositol turnover on differentiation of some human myelomonocytic leukemia cells. *Leukemia Res* 15(8): 701.

199. Makishima, M. et al. 1993. Differentiation of human monoblastic leukemia U937 cells induced by inhibitors of myosin light chain kinase and prevention of differentiation by granulocyte-macrophage colony-stimulating factor. *Biochim Biophys Acta* 1176(3): 245-249.

200. Mallett, A. K. et al. 1987. Dietary modification of intestinal bacterial enzyme activities--potential formation of toxic agents in the gut. *Scand J Gastroenterol Suppl* 129: 251-257.

201. Markkanen, T. et al. 1981. Antiherpetic agent from juniper tree (Juniperus communis), its purification, identification, and testing in primary human amnion cell cultures. *Drugs Exp Clin Res* 7: 691-697.

202. Marks, D. R. et al. 1993. A double-blind placebo-controlled trial of intranasal capsaicin for cluster headache. *Cephalalgia* 13(2): 114-116.

203. Martin, P. M. et al., 1978. Phytoestrogen interaction with estrogen receptors in human breast cancer cells. *Endocrinology* 103(5): 1860-1867.

204. Matheson, H. B. et al. 1995. Cholesterol 7-a-hydroxylase activity is increased by dietary modification with psyllium hydrocolloid, pectin, cholesterol, and cholestyramine in rats. *J Nutr* 125(3): 454-458.

205. Matos, O. C. et al. 1999. Sensitivity of Fusarium strains to Chelidonium majus L. extracts. *J Ethnopharmacol* 66(2): 151-158.

206. Matsukawa, Y. et al. 1993. Genistein arrests cell cycle progression at G2-M. *Cancer Res* 53(6): 1328-1331.

207. Mazur, A. et al. 1991. Apolipoprotein B gene expression in rat intestine. The effect of dietary fiber. FEBS *Lett* 284(1): 63-65.

208. McGuffin, M. et al. 1997. American Herbal Products Association's Botanical Safety Handbook. Boca Raton, FL: CRC Press.

209. McKevoy, G. K. (ed.). 1998. AHFS Drug Information. Bethesda, MD: American Society of Health-System Pharmacists.

210. Meehan, A. G. and D. L. Kreulen. 1992. A capsaicin-sensitive inhibitory reflex from the colon to mesenteric arteries in the guinea-pig. *J Physiol* 448: 153-159.

211. Melnyk, A. and J. Himms-Hagen. 1995. Resistance to aging-associated obesity in capsaicin-desensitized rats one year after treatment. *Obes Res* 3(4): 337-344.

212. Menke, J. J. and J. R. Heins. 1999. Treatment of postherpetic neuralgia. *J Am Pharm Assoc* (Wash) 39(2): 217-221.

213. Meydani, M. et al. 1998. The effect of long-term dietary supplementation with antioxidants. *Ann NY Acad Sci* 854: 352-360.

214. Miksicek, R. J. 1994. Interaction of naturally occurring nonsteroidal estrogens with expressed recombinant human estrogen receptor. *J Steroid Biochem Mol Biol* 49(2-3): 152-160.

215. Miller, M. S. et al. 1983. Interaction of capsaicinoids with drug metabolizing systems: Relationship to toxicity. *Biochem Pharmacol* 32: 547-551.

216. Mills, S. 1994. The Complete Guide to Modern Herbalism. Great Britain: Thorsons.

217. Miyake, T. et al. 1998. Possible inhibition of atherosclerosis by a flavonoid isolated from young green barley leaves. In Shibamoto, T. et al. (eds.). Functional foods for disease prevention II. Washington, DC: American Chemical Society.

218. Modly, C. E. et al. 1986. Capsaicin as an in vitro inhibitor of benzo[a]pyrene metabolism and its DNA binding in human and murine keratinocytes. *Drug Metab Dispos* 14: 413-417.

219. Molina-Torres, J. et al. 1999. Antimicrobial properties of alkamides present in flavouring plants traditionally used in Mesoamerica: affinin and capsaicin. *J Ethnopharmacol* 64(3): 241-248.

220. Monsereenusorn, Y. 1983. Subchronic toxicity studies of capsaicin and capsicum in rats. *Res Commun Chem Pathol Pharmacol* 41(1): 95-110.

221. Montanini, I. et al. 1977. The effect of silybin on liver phospholipid synthesis in the rat in vivo. *Farmaco* [Sci] 32(2): 141-146.

222. Morita, K. et al. 1984. A desmutagenic factor isolated from burdock (Arctium lappa Linne). *Mutat Res* 129(1): 25-31.

223. Moritani, S. et al. 1996. Cytotoxic components of bardanae fructus (goboshi). Biol Pharm Bull 19(11): 1515-1517.

224. Morre, D. J. et al. 1995. Capsaicin inhibits preferentially the NADH oxidase and growth of transformed cells in culture. *Proc Natl Acad Sci USA* 92(6): 1831-1835.

225. Morre, D. J. et al. 1996. Capsaicin inhibits plasma membrane NADH oxidase and growth of human and mouse melanoma lines. *Eur J Cancer* 32A(11): 1995-2003.

226. Morton, M. S. et al. 1994. Determination of lignans and isoflavonoids in human female plasma following dietary supplementation. *J Endocrinol* 142(2): 251-259.

227. Moss, R. W. 1992. Cancer Therapy: The Independent Consumer's Guide to Non-Toxic Treatment and Prevention. New York: Equinox.

Monographs

References

228. Mousavi, Y. and H. Adlercreutz. 1992. Enterolactone and estradiol inhibit each other's proliferative effect on MCF-7 breast cancer cells in culture. *J Steroid Biochem Mol Biol* 41(3-8): 615-619.

229. Mousavi, Y. and H. Adlercreutz. 1993. Genistein is an effective stimulator of sex hormone-binding globulin production in hepatocarcinoma human liver cancer cells and suppresses proliferation of these cells in culture. *Steroids* 58(7): 301-304.

230. Nadkarni, K. M. 1976. Indian Materia Medica. Bombay: Popular Prakashan. 268-271.

231. Nagashima, K. 1989. Inhibitory effect of eugenol on Cu2+ catalysed lipid peroxidation in human erythrocyte membrane. *Int J Biochem* 21: 745-749.

232. Naim, M. et al. 1976. Antioxidative and antihemolytic activities of soybean isoflavones. *J Agric Food Chem* 24(6): 1174-1177.

233. Nassuato, G. et al. 1991. Effect of silibinin on biliary lipid composition: Experimental and clinical study. *J Hepatol* 12(3): 290-295.

234. NCI: National Cancer Institute, US Department of Health and Human Services. 1985. Diet, nurtition, and cancer prevention: A guide to food choices. DHHS Pub No. NIH 85-2711. Washington, DC: US Government Printing Office.

235. Nestel, P. J. et al. 1999. Isoflavones from red clover improve systemic arterial compliance but not plasma lipids in menopausal women. *J Clin Endocrinol Metab* 84(3):895-898.

236. Nestle, M. 1998. Broccoli sprouts in cancer prevention. *Nutr Rev* 56(4 Pt 1): 127-130.

237. Newall, C. A. et al. 1996. Herbal Medicine: A Guide for Healthcare Professionals. London, UK: The Pharmaceutical Press.

238. Nijhoff, W. A. 1995. Effects of consumption of Brussels sprouts on intestinal and lymphocytic glutathione-S-transferases in humans. *Carcinogenesis* 16(9): 2125-2128.

239. Nishino, H. et al. 1999. Suppression of lung and liver carcinogenesis in mice by oral administration of myo-inositol. *Anticancer Res* 19(5A): 3663-3664.

240. Nolano, M. et al. 1999. Topical capsaicin in humans: parallel loss of epidermal nerve fibers and pain sensation. *Pain* 81(1-2): 135-145.

241. Nordgaard, I. et al. 1996. Colonic production of butyrate in patients with previous colonic cancer during long-term treatment with dietary fiber (Plantago ovata seeds). *Scand J Gastroenterol* 31(10): 1011-1020.

242. Nowicky, J. W. et al. 1991. Evaluation of thiophosphoric acid alkaloid derivatives from Chelidonium majus L. ("Ukrain") as an immunostimulant in patients with various carcinomas. *Drugs Exp Clin Res* 17(2): 139-143.

243. Nwannenna A. I. et al. 1994. Effects of oestrogenic silage on some clinical and endocrinological parameters in ovariectomized heifers. *Acta Vet Scand* 35(2): 173-183.

244. Nwannenna A. I. et al. 1995. Clinical changes in ovariectomized ewes exposed to phytoestrogens and 17 b-estradiol implants. *Proc Soc Exp Biol Med* 208(1): 92-97.

245. Ohkami, H. et al. 1995. Effects of apple pectin on fecal bacterial enzymes in azoxymethane-induced rat colon carcinogenesis. *Jpn J Cancer Res* 86(6): 523-529.

246. Okura, A. et al. 1988. Effect of genistein on topoisomerase activity and on the growth of [Val 12]Ha-ras-transformed NIH 3T3 cells. *Biochem Biophys Res Commun* 157(1): 183-189.

247. Osborn, R. W. et al. 1995. Isolation and characterization of plant defensins from seeds of Asteraceae, Fabaceae, Hippocastanaceae, and Saxifragaceae. *FEBS Lett* 368(2): 257-262.

248. Palasciano, G. et al. 1994. The effect of silymarin on plasma levels of malondialdehyde in patients receiving long-term treatment with psychotropic drugs. *Curr Ther Res* 55:537-545.

249. Palevitch, D. and L. E. Craker. 1995. Nutritional and Medical Importance of Red Pepper (Capsicum spp.). *J Herbs Spices Med Plants* 3(2): 55-83.

250. Panzer, A. et al. 2000. The antimitotic effects of Ukrain, a Chelidonium majus alkaloid derivative, are reversible in vitro. *Cancer Lett* 150(1): 85-92.

251. Perera, M. I. et al. 1987. Free radical injury and liver tumor promotion. *Toxicol Pathol* 15(1): 51-59.

252. Peskar, B. M. et al. 1995. Functional ablation of sensory neurons impairs healing of acute gastric mucosal damage in rats. *Dig Dis Sci* 40(11): 2460-2464.

253. Peterson, G. and S. Barnes. 1991. Genistein inhibition of the growth of human breast cancer cells: Independence from estrogen receptors and the multi-drug resistance gene. *Biochem Biophys Res Commun* 179(1): 661-667.

254. Peterson, G. and S. Barnes. 1993. Genistein and biochanin A inhibit the growth of human prostate cancer cells but not epidermal growth factor receptor tyrosine autophosphorylation. *Prostate* 22(4): 335-345.

255. Petit, P. et al. 1993. Effects of a fenugreek seed extract on feeding behavior in the rat: Metabolic-endocrine correlates. *Pharmacol Biochem Behav* 45(2): 369-374.

256. Petit, P. R. et al. 1995. Steroid saponins from fenugreek seeds: Extraction, purification, and pharmacological investigation on feeding behavior and plasma cholesterol. *Steroids* 60(10): 674-680.

257. Pieri, C. et al. 1990. Antioxidant enzymes in erythrocytes from old and diet restricted old rats. *Boll Soc Ital Biol Sper* 66(10): 909-914.

258. Pietrangelo, A. et al. 1995. Molecular and cellular aspects of iron-induced hepatic cirrhosis in rodents. *J Clin Invest* 95(4): 1824-1831.

259. Pizzorno, J. E. and M. T. Murray (Eds.). 1999. Textbook of Natural Medicine, Vol. 2. Edinburgh: Harcourt Publishers Limited. 1128, 1131.

260. Platel, K. and K. Srinivasan. 2000. Influence of dietary spices and their active principles on pancreatic digestive enzymes in albino rats. *Nahrung* 44(1): 42-46.

261. Prochaska, H. J. et al. 1992. Rapid detection of inducers of enzymes that protect against carcinogens. *Proc Natl Acad Sci USA* 89(6): 2394-2398.

262. Pulla Reddy, A. C. and B. R. Lokesh. 1992. Studies on spice principles as antioxidants in the inhibition of lipid peroxidation of rat liver microsomes. *Mol Cell Biochem* 111(1-2): 117-124.

263. Pulla Reddy, A. C. and B. R. Lokesh. 1994. Studies on the inhibitory effects of curcumin and eugenol on the formation of reactive oxygen species and the oxidation of ferrous iron. *Mol Cell Biochem* 137: 1-8.

264. Quettier-Deleu, C. et al. 2000. Phenolic compounds and antioxidant activities of buckwheat (Fagopyrum esculentum Moench) hulls and flour. *J Ethnopharmacol* 72(1-2): 35-42.

265. Rao, G. et al. 1990. Effect of dietary restriction on the age-dependent changes in the expression of antioxidant enzymes in rat liver. *J Nutr* 120(6): 602-609.

266. Ravikumar, P. and C. V. Anuradha. 1999. Effect of fenugreek seeds on blood lipid peroxidation and antioxidants in diabetic rats. *Phytother Res* 13(3): 197-201.

267. Regal, J. F. et al. 2000. Dietary phytoestrogens have anti-inflammatory activity in a guinea pig model of asthma. *Proc Soc Exp Biol Med* 223(4): 372-378.

268. Reinhart, K. C. et al. 1999. Xeno-oestrogens and phyto-oestrogens induce the synthesis of leukaemia inhibitory factor by human and bovine oviduct cells. *Mol Hum Reprod* 5(10): 899-907.

269. Rhoads, P. M. et al. 1984-85. Anticholinergic poisonings associated with commercial burdock root tea. *J Toxicol Clin Toxicol* 22(6): 581-584.

270. Rigaud, D. et al. 1998. Effect of psyllium on gastric emptying, hunger feeling and food intake in normal volunteers: A double blind study. *Eur J Clin Nutr* 52(4): 239-245.

271. Robbers, J. E. and V. E. Tyler. 1999. Tyler's Herbs of Choice. Binghamton, NY: Hawthorn Herbal Press.

272. Rodriguez, P. et al. 1995. Allergic contact dermatitis due to burdock (Arctium lappa). *Contact Dermatitis* 33(2): 134-135.

273. Roncucci, L. et al. 1998. Aberrant crypt foci in patients with colorectal cancer. *Br J Cancer* 77(12): 2343-2348.

274. Ruiz-Larrea, M. B. et al. 1997. Antioxidant activity of phytoestrogenic isoflavones. *Free Radic Res* 26(1): 63-70.

275. Rushmore, T. H. et al. 1984. Rapid lipid peroxidation in the nuclear fraction of rat liver induced by a diet deficient in choline and methionine. *Cancer Lett* 24(3): 251-255.

276. Rushmore, T. H. et al. 1986. A choline-devoid diet, carcinogenic in the rat, induces DNA damage and repair. *Carcinogenesis* 7(10): 1677-1680.

277. Sadzuka, Y. et al. 1997. Protective effect of flavonoids on dioxorubicin-induced cardiotoxicity Toxicology Lett 92(1): 1-7.

278. Saito, A. et al. 1999. Effects of capsaicin on serum triglycerides and free fatty acid in olive oil treated rats. *Int J Vitam Nutr Res* 69(5): 337-340.

279. Salimath, B. P. and M. N. Satyanarayana. 1987. Inhibition of calcium and calmodulin-dependent phosphodiesterase activity in rats by capsaicin. *Biochem Biophys Res Commun* 148(1): 292-299.

280. Salmi, H. A. and S. Sarna. 1982. Effect of silymarin on chemical, functional, and morphological alterations of the liver. A double-blind controlled study. *Scand J Gastroenterol* 17(4): 517-521.

281. Sambaiah, K. and M. N. Satyanarayana. 1980. Hypocholesterolemic effect of red pepper and capsaicin. *Indian J Exp Biol* 18(8): 898-899.

282. Sanchez de Medina, F. et al. 1994. Hypoglycemic activity of juniper "berries." *Planta Med* 60(3): 197-200.

283. Sarkar, D. et al. 1994. Chlorophyll and chlorophyllin as modifiers of genotoxic effects. *Mutat Res* 318(3): 239-247.

284. Sauvaire, Y. et al. 1998. 4-hydroxyisoleucine: A novel amino acid potentiator of insulin secretion. *Diabetes* 47(2): 206-210.

285. Savitha, G. et al. 1990. Capsaicin inhibits calmodulin-mediated oxidative burst in rat macrophages. *Cell Signal* 2(6): 577-585.

286. Schweigerer, L. et al. 1992. Identification in human urine of a natural growth inhibitor for cells derived from solid paediatric tumours. *Eur J Clin Invest* 22(4): 260-264.

287. Sievers, A.F. 1930. The Herb Hunters Guide. Misc. Publ. No. 77. USDA, Washington DC.

288. Serraino, M. and L. U. Thompson. 1991. The effect of flaxseed supplementation on early risk markers for mammary carcinogenesis. *Cancer Lett* 60: 135-142.

289. Serraino, M. and L. U. Thompson. 1992a. Flaxseed supplementation and early markers of colon carcinogenesis. *Cancer Lett* 63: 159-165.

290. Serraino, M. and L. U. Thompson. 1992b. The effect of flaxseed supplementation on the initiation and promotional stages of mammary tumorigenesis. *Nutr Cancer* 17(2): 153-159.

291. Severson, R. K. et al. 1989. A prospective study of demographics, diet, and prostate cancer among men of Japanese ancestry in Hawaii. *Cancer Res* 49(7): 1857-1860.

292. Shamsuddin, A. M. et al. 1997. IP6: A novel anti-cancer agent. *Life Sci* 61(4): 343-354.

293. Sharma, R. D. 1979. Isoflavones and hypercholesterolemia in rats. *Lipids* 14(6): 535-539.

294. Sharma, R. D. et al. 1990. Effect of fenugreek seeds on blood glucose and serum lipids in Type I diabetes. *Eur J Clin Nutr* 44(4): 301-306.

295. Sharma, O. P. et al. 1992. Soy of dietary source plays a preventive role against the pathogenesis of prostatitis in rats. *J Steroid Biochem Mol Biol* 43(6): 557-564.

296. Shih-Chen, L. et al. 1973. Chinese Medicinal Herbs. San Francisco, CA: Georgetown Press.

297. Shimoi, K. et al. 1997. Protection by (alpha) G-Rutin, a water-soluble antioxidant flavonoid, against renal damage in mice treated with ferric nitrilotriacetate. *J Cancer Res* 88(5): 453-460.

298. Shronts, E. P. 1997. Essential nature of choline with implications for total parenteral nutrition. *J Am Diet Assoc* 97(6): 639-646, 649.

299. Sicuteri, F. et al. 1990. Substance P theory: A unique focus on the painful and painless phenomena of cluster headache. *Headache* 30(2): 69-79.

300. Simic, M. G. and D. S. Bergtold. 1991. Dietary modulation of DNA damage in human. *Mutat Res* 250(1-2): 17-24.

301. Slaga, T. J. et al. 1981. Skin tumor-promoting activity of benzoyl peroxide, a widely used free radical-generating compound. *Science* 213(4511): 1023-1025.

302. Slattery, M. L. et al. 1997. Are dietary factors involved in DNA methylation associated with colon cancer? *Nutr Cancer* 28(1): 52-62.

303. Slattery, M. L. et al. 2000. Interplay between dietary inducers of GST and the GSTM-1 genotype in colon cancer. *Int J Cancer* 87(5): 728-733.

304. Slavin, J. L. 1999. Implementation of dietary modifications. *Am J Med* 106(1A): 46S-51S.

305. Sohal, R. S. et al. 1994. Oxidative damage, mitochondrial oxidant generation, and antioxidant defenses during aging and in response to food restriction in the mouse. *Mech Ageing Dev* 74(1-2): 121-133.

306. Sotomayor, E. M. et al. 1992. Enhancement of macrophage tumouricidal activity by the alkaloid derivative Ukrain. In vitro and in vivo studies. *Drugs Exp Clin Res* 18 Suppl: 5-11.

307. Sprecher, D. L. et al. 1993. Efficacy of psyllium in reducing serum cholesterol levels in hypercholesterolemic patients on high– or low-fat diets. *Ann Intern Med* 119(7 Pt 1): 545-554.

308. Srinivasan, M. R. and M. N. Satyanarayana. 1989. Effect of capsaicin on skeletal muscle lipoprotein lipase in rats fed high fat diet. *Indian J Exp Biol* 27(10): 910-912.

309. Staack, R. et al. 1998. A comparison of the individual and collective effects of four glucosinolate breakdown products from brussels sprouts on induction of detoxification enzymes. *Toxicol Appl Pharmacol.* 149(1): 17-23.

310. Stanberry, L. R. et al. 1992. Capsaicin-sensitive peptidergic neurons are involved in the zosteriform spread of herpes simplex virus infection. *J Med Virol* 38(2): 142-146.

311. Stark, A. and Z. Madar. 1993. The effect of an ethanol extract derived from fenugreek (Trigonella foenum-graecum) on bile acid absorption and cholesterol levels in rats. *Br J Nutr* 69(1): 277-287.

312. Steinacker, J. et al. 1996. Ukrain therapy in a frontal anaplastic grade III astrocytoma (case report). *Drugs Exp Clin Res* 22(3-5): 275-277.

313. Steinbach, G. et al. 1994. Effect of caloric restriction on colonic proliferation in obese persons: implications for colon cancer prevention. *Cancer Res* 54(5): 1194-1197.

314. Steinmetz, K. A. et al. 1993. Vegetables, fruit, and lung cancer in the Iowa Women's Health Study. *Cancer Res* 53(3): 536-543.

315. Su, S. J. et al. 2000. The potential of soybean foods as a chemoprevention approach for human urinary tract cancer. *Clin Cancer Res* 6(1): 230-236.

316. Surh, Y. J. et al. 1995. Chemoprotective effects of capsaicin and diallyl sulfide against mutagenesis or tumorigenesis by vinyl carbamate and N-nitrosodimethylamine. *Carcinogenesis* 16(10): 2467-2471.

317. Surh, Y. J. et al. 1998. Chemoprotective properties of some pungent ingredients present in red pepper and ginger. *Mutat Res* 402(1-2): 259-267.

318. Swanston-Flatt, S. K. 1989. Glycaemic effects of traditional European plant treatments for diabetes. Studies in normal and streptozotocin diabetic mice. *Diabetes Res* 10(2): 69-73.

319. Swantston-Flatt, S. K. et al. 1990. Traditional plant treatments for diabetes. Studies in normal and streptozotocin diabetic mice. *Diabetologia* 33(8): 462-464.

320. Taber, C. W. 1962. Taber's Cyclopedic Medical Dictionary, 9th ed. Philadelphia: F. A. Davis Company. C-11.

321. Takayama, T. et al. 1998. Aberrant crypt foci of the colon as precursors of adenoma and cancer. *N Engl J Med* 339(18): 1277-1284.

322. Takeda, Y. et al. 1992. Reversal of multidrug resistance by tyrosine-kinase inhibitors in a non-P-glycoprotein-mediated multidrug-resistant cell line. *Int J Cancer* 57(2): 229-239.

323. Tavani, A. 1996. Food and nutrition intake and risk of cataract. *Ann Epidemiol* 6(1): 41-46.

324. Tawfiq, N. et al. 1994. Induction of the anti-carcinogenic enzyme quinone reductase by food extracts using murine hepatoma cells. *Eur J Cancer Prev* 3(3): 285-292.

325. Tazawa, K. et al. 1997. Anticarcinogenic action of apple pectin on fecal enzyme activities and mucosal or portal prostaglandin E2 levels in experimental rat colon carcinogenesis. *J Exp Clin Cancer Res* 16(1): 33-38.

326. Tazawa, K. et al. 1999. Dietary fiber inhibits the incidence of hepatic metastasis with the antioxidant activity and portal scavenging functions. *Hum Cell* 12(4): 189-196.

327. Teel, R. W. 1991. Effects of capsaicin on rat liver S9-mediated metabolism and DNA binding of aflatoxin. *Nutr Cancer* 15(1): 27-32.

328. Teel, R. W. 1993. Effect of phytochemicals on the mutagenicity of the tobacco-specific nitrosamine 4-(methylnitrosamino)-1-(3-pyridyl)-1-butanone (NNK) in Salmonella typhimurium strain TA1535. *Phytother Res* 7: 248-251.

329. Teel, R. et al. 1997. Effects of capsaicin on the metabolic activation of heterocyclic amines and on cytochrome P450 1A2 activity in hamster liver microsomes. *Proc Am Assoc Cancer Res* 38: 363.

330. Teng, C. H. et al. 1998. Protective action of capsaicin and chilli on haemorrhagic shock-induced gastric mucosal injury in the rat. *J Gastroenterol Hepatol* 13(10): 1007-1014.

331. Terras, F. R. et al. 1992. Analysis of two novel classes of plant antifungal proteins from radish (Raphanus sativus L.). *J Biol Chem* 267(22): 15301-15309.

332. Thevissen, K. et al. 1997. Specific, high affinity binding sites for an antifungal plant defensin on Neurospora crassa hyphae and microsomal membranes. *J Biol Chem* 272(51): 32176-32181.

333. Thompson, L. U. and M. Serraino. 1990. Lignans in flaxseed and breast and colon carcinogenesis. In: Proceedings of the Flax Institute of the U.S., January 25-26. Fargo, North Dakota. 30-35.

334. Toda, S. and Y. Shirataki. 1999. Inhibitory effects of isoflavones on lipid peroxidation by reactive oxygen species. *Phytother Res* 13(2): 163-165.

335. Tomotake, H. et al. 2000. A buckwheat protein product suppresses gallstone formation and plasma cholesterol more strongly than soy protein isolate in hamsters. *J Nutr* 130(7): 1670-1674.

336. Traganos, F. et al. 1992. Effects of genistein on the growth and cell cycle progression of normal human lymphocytes and human leukemic MOLT-4 and HL-60 cells. *Cancer Res* 52(22): 6200-6208.

337. Trautwein, E. A. et al. 1999. Increased fecal bile acid excretion and changes in the circulating bile acid pool are involved in the hypocholesterolemic and gall-stone preventive actions of psyllium in hamsters. *J Nutr* 129(4): 896-902.

338. Tyler, V. E. 1993. The Honest Herbal. Binghamton, NY: Pharmaceutical Products Press. 219-220.

339. Tyler, V. E. 1994. Herbs of Choice. Binghamton, NY: Pharmaceutical Products Press.

340. Umehara, K. et al. 1996. Studies on differentiation inducers. VI. Lignan derivatives from Arctium fructus (2). *Chem Pharm Bull* (Tokyo) 44(12): 2300-2304.

341. Vahlensieck, U. et al. 1995. The effect of Chelidonium majus herb extract on choleresis in the isolated perfused rat liver. *Planta Med* 61(3): 267-271.

342. Valenzuela, A. et al. 1989. Selectivity of silymarin on the increase of the glutathione content in different tissues of the rat. *Planta Med* 55(5): 420-422.

343. Valenzuela, A. and A. Garrido. 1994. Biochemical bases of the pharmacological action of the flavonoid silymarin and of its structural isomer silibinin. *Biol Res* 27(2): 105-112.

344. Vanner, S. 1993. Mechanism of action of capsaicin on submucosal arterioles in the guinea pig ileum. *Am J Physiol* 265(1 Pt 1): G51-55.

345. Vanner, S. 1994. Corelease of neuropeptides from capsaicin-sensitive afferents dilates submucosal arterioles in guinea pig ileum. *Am J Physiol* 267(4 Pt 1): G650-655.

346. van Poppel, G. et al. 1999. Brassica vegetables and cancer prevention: Epidemiology and mechanisms. *Adv Exp Med Biol* 472: 159-168.

347. Vaswani, S. K. et al. 1996. Psyllium laxative-induced anaphylaxis, asthma, and rhinitis. *Allergy* 51(4): 266-268.

348. Vazquez-Olivencia, W. et al. 1992. The effect of red and black pepper on orocecal transit time. *J Am Coll Nutr* 11(2): 228-231.

349. Verhagen, H. et al. 1995. Reduction of oxidative DNA-damage in humans by Brussels sprouts. *Carcinogenesis* 16(4): 969-970.

350. Verhoeven, D. T. et al. 1996. Epidemiological studies on brassica vegetables and cancer risk. *Cancer Epidemiol Biomarkers Prev* 5(9): 733-748.

351. Verma, S. P. and B. R. Goldin. 1998. Effect of soy-derived isoflavonoids on the induced growth of MCF-7 cells by estrogenic environmental chemicals. *Nutr Cancer* 30(3): 232-239.

352. Vermeulen, E. G. et al. 2000. Effect of homocysteine-lowering treatment with folic acid plus vitamin B6 on progression of subclinical atherosclerosis: A randomised, placebo-controlled trial. *Lancet* 355(9203): 517-522.

353. Versantvoort, C. H. et al. 1993. Genistein modulates the decreased drug accumulation in non-P-glycoprotein mediated multidrug resistant tumour cells. *Br J Cancer* 68(5): 939-946.

354. Visudhiphan, S. et al. 1982. The relationship between high fibrinolytic activity and daily capsicum ingestion in Thais. *Am J Clin Nutr* 35(6): 1452-1458.

355. Voltchek, I. V. et al. 1996. Potential therapeutic efficacy of Ukrain (NSC 631570) in AIDS patients with Kaposi's sarcoma. *Drugs Exp Clin Res* 22(3-5): 283-286.

356. Voorrips, L. E. et al. 2000. Vegetable and fruit consumption and lung cancer risk in the Netherlands Cohort Study on diet and cancer. *Cancer Causes Control* 11(2): 101-115.

357. Walford, R. L. et al. 1999. Physiologic changes in humans subjected to severe, selective calorie restriction for two years in Biosphere 2: Health, aging, and toxicological perspectives. *Toxicological Sciences* 52(2 Suppl.): 61-65.

358. Walters, R. 1993. Options: The Alternative Cancer Therapy Book. Garden City Park, NY: Avery Publishing Group.

359. Wang, C. and M. S. Kurzer. 1997. Phytoestrogen concentration determines effects on DNA synthesis in human breast cancer cells. *Nutr Cancer* 28(3): 236-247.

360. Wang, W. et al. 1998. Induction of NADPH:quinone reductase by dietary phytoestrogens in Colonic Colo205 cells. *Biochem Pharmacol* 56(2): 189-195.

361. Wargovich, M. J. et al. 2000. Efficacy of potential chemopreventive agents on rat colon aberrant crypt formation and progression. *Carcinogenesis* 21(6): 1149-1155.

362. Watanabe, T. et al. 1987. Capsaicin, a pungent principle of hot red pepper, evokes catecholamine secretion from the adrenal medulla of anesthetized rats. *Biochem Biophys Res Commun* 142(1): 259-264.

363. Watanabe, T. et al. 1989. Inhibitors for protein-tyrosine kinases, ST638 and genistein: induce differentiation of mouse erythroleukemia cells in a synergistic manner. *Exp Cell Res* 183(2): 335-342.

364. Watanabe, S. and S. Koessel. 1993. Colon cancer: An approach from molecular epidemiology. *J Epidemiol* 3: 47-61.

365. Watson, C. P. et al. 1993. A randomized vehicle-controlled trial of topical capsaicin in the treatment of postherpetic neuralgia. *Clin Ther* 15(3): 510-526.

366. Wei, H. et al. 1993. Inhibition of tumor promoter-induced hydrogen peroxide formation in vitro and in vivo by genistein. *Nutr Cancer* 20(1): 1-12.

367. Wei, H. et al. 1996. Inhibition of UV light– and Fenton reaction-induced oxidative DNA damage by the soybean isoflavone genistein. *Carcinogenesis* 17(1): 73-77.

368. Weindruch, R. 1992. Effect of caloric restriction on age-associated cancers. *Exp Gerontol* 27(5-6): 575-581.

369. Weindruch, R. 1996. Caloric restriction and aging. *Scientific American* 274(1): 32-38.

370. Whistler, W.A. 1992. Polynesian Herbal Medicine. Lawai, Kauai, Hawaii: National Tropical Botanical Garden. 237.

371. Widyarini, S. et al. 2000. Protective effect of isoflavone derivative against photocarcinogenesis in a mouse model. *Redox Rep* 5(2-3):156-158.

372. Wolever, T. M. et al. 1994. Method of administration influences the serum cholesterol-lowering effect of psyllium. *Am J Clin Nutr* 59(5): 1055-1059.

373. Wolvetang, E. J. 1996. Apoptosis induced by inhibitors of the plasma membrane NADH-oxidase involves Bcl-2 and calcineurin. Cell Growth Differ 7(10): 1315-1325.

374. Wood, A.B. 1987. Determination of the pungent principles of chilies and ginger by reversed-phase high-performance liquid chromatography with use of a single standard substance. *Flavour Fragrance J* 2: 1–12.

375. Xian, M. S. et al. 1989. Efficacy of traditional Chinese herbs on squamous cell carcinoma of the esophagus: histopathologic analysis of 240 cases. *Acta Med Okayama* 43(6): 345-351.

376. Yanagihara, K. et al. 1993. Antiproliferative effects of isoflavones on human cancer cell lines established from the gastrointestinal tract. *Cancer Res* 53(23): 5815-5821.

377. Yeoh, K. G. et al. 1995. Chili protects against aspirin-induced gastroduodenal mucosal injury in humans. *Dig Dis Sci* 40(3): 580-583.

378. Yin, F. et al. 1999. Growth inhibitory effects of flavonoids in human thyroid cancer cell lines. *Thyroid* 9(4): 369-376.

379. Yoshioka, M. et al. 1995. Effects of red-pepper diet on the energy metabolism in men. *J Nutr Sci Vitaminol* (Tokyo) 41(6): 647-656.

380. Yu, B. P. 1993. Antioxidant action of dietary restriction in the aging process. *J Nutr Sci Vitaminol* (Tokyo) 39 Suppl: S75-S83.

381. Yu, B. P. 1996. Aging and oxidative stress: Modulation by dietary restriction. *Free Radic Biol Med* 21(5): 651-668.

382. Yu, B. P. 1999. Approaches to anti-aging intervention: The promises and the uncertainties. *Mech Ageing Dev* 111(2-3): 73-87.

383. Yu, R. et al. 1998. Modulation of select immune responses by dietary capsaicin. *Int J Vitam Nutr Res* 68(2): 114-119.

384. Yun, C-H. et al. 1995. Non-specific inhibition of cytochrome P450 activities by chlorophyllin in human and rat liver microsomes. *Carcinogenesis* 16(6): 1437-1440.

385. Zand, R. S. et al. 2000. Steroid hormone activity of flavonoids and related compounds. *Breast Cancer Res Treat* 62(1): 35-49.

386. Zava, D. T. et al. 1998. Estrogen and progestin bioactivity of foods, herbs, and spices. *Proc Soc Exp Biol Med* 217(3): 369-378.

387. Zeisel, S. H. et al. 1991. Choline, an essential nutrient for humans. *FASEB J* 5(7): 2093-2098.

388. Zeisel, S. H. 1992. Choline: an important nutrient in brain development, liver function and carcinogenesis. *J Am Coll Nutr* 11(5): 473-481.

389. Zhang, Y. et al. 1992. A major inducer of anticarcinogenic protective enzymes from broccoli: Isolation and elucidation of structure. *Proc Natl Acad Sci USA* 89(6): 2399-2403.

390. Zhang, Y. et al. 1994. Anticarcinogenic activities of sulphoraphane and structurally related synthetic norbornyl isothiocyanates. *Proc Natl Acad Sci USA* 91(8): 3147-3150.

391. Zhang, Z. et al. 1993. Inhibition of liver microsomal cytochrome P450 activity and metabolism of the tobacco-specific nitrosamine NNK by capsaicin and ellagic acid. *Anticancer Res* 13(6A): 2341-2346.

392. Zhang, Z. et al. 1997. Effects of orally administered capsaicin, the principle component of capsicum fruits, on the in vitro metabolism of the tobacco-specific nitrosamine NNK in hamster lung and liver microsomes. *Anticancer Res* 17(2A): 1093-1098.

393. Zhu, Z. et al. 1997. Effect of caloric restriction on pre-malignant and malignant stages of mammary carcinogenesis. *Carcinogenesis* 18(5): 1007-1012.

394. Zi, X. et al. 1997. Novel cancer chemopreventive effects of a flavonoid antioxidant silymarin: inhibition of mRNA expression of an endogenous tumor promoter TNFa. *Biochem Biophys Res Commun* 239(1): 334-339.

395. Zi, X. et al. 1998a. A flavonoid antioxidant, silymarin, inhibits activation of erbB1 signaling and induces cyclin-dependent kinase inhibitors, G1 arrest, and anticarcinogenic effects in human prostate carcinoma DU145 cells. *Cancer Res* 58(9): 1920-1929.

396. Zi, X. et al. 1998b. Anticarcinogenic effect of a flavonoid antioxidant, silymarin, in human breast cancer cells MDA-MB 468: induction of G1 arrest through an increase in Cip1/p21 concomitant with a decrease in kinase activity of cyclin-dependent kinases and associated cyclins. *Clin Cancer Res* 4(4): 1055-1064.

397. Zi, X. and R. Agarwal. 1999. Silibinin decreases prostate-specific antigen with cell growth inhibition via G1 arrest, leading to differentiation of prostate carcinoma cells: implications for prostate cancer intervention. *Proc Natl Acad Sci USA* 96(13): 7490-7495.

PART 3

COMPLIMENTARY METHODS
OF PURIFICATION

"The art of medicine consists in amusing the patient while nature cures the disease."
—Voltaire

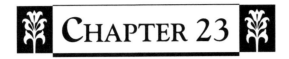

CHAPTER 23

DIET & EXERCISE

"It is a very odd thing-
As odd as can be-
That whatever Miss T. eats
Turns into Miss T."
–De La Mare

23
⇒⟫✳⟪⇐

Diet & Exercise

23.1 Diet

The herbs and foods detailed in the scientific monographs are valuable tools that can aid the body in carrying out the purification process, particularly when they are taken together in synergistic, alchemic formulas aimed at nourishing the body and encouraging the elimination of toxins. Equally important to the process is the incorporation of daily eating habits that readily shift ones dynamic internal mechanisms towards creating an optimum state of health. Included in this book are three recommended 21-day programs that include a diet and supplement regimen that will help the body to successfully carry out the purification process. The dietary suggestions vary depending on the physical, mental, emotional and spiritual levels of each individual, and the level of purification that he/she is ready to experience. However, all of the nutritional recommendations stem from the following list of 16 vital dietary principles to live by for optimal health. In Appendix B practitioners will find a quick list to share with patients of the 16 principles described below. Incorporating these practices into one's daily life, even beyond the 21-day purification process, is a powerful way to create a new, health-giving physical body that will support a clearer, more balanced mental, emotional, and spiritual body.

16 Vital Principles to Live by for Optimal Health

1. Avoid eating if you feel stressed or anxious.

2. Listen to your body - don't eat if you're not hungry, and conversely, don't put up with hunger pains. Stop eating once you begin to feel full and no longer have an appetite.

3. Drink 8 to 12 glasses of filtered water daily. Avoid large amounts of fluid with meals.

4. Avoid eating large amounts of sugar - especially refined sugars.

5. Avoid caffeine.

6. Avoid foods you may be allergic to.

7. Chew your food slowly.

8. Limit your intake, and if possible avoid packaged and processed foods containing artificial chemicals such as preservatives, colorings, flavorings and synthetic sweeteners.

9. Try to eat organically grown fresh produce, free of pesticides and herbicides.

10. Try to eat organically-reared animal products, stay clear of reheated meats and always buy free-range eggs.

11. Obtain your protein from diverse sources (including legumes) not just from animal products such as meat, eggs and fish - you can obtain first-class protein by combining in one meal any three of the four following foods - grains (wheat, buckwheat, rice, barley, rye, oats, millet etc.), nuts, seeds and legumes.

12. Choose your breads wisely - it is important to eat only good quality breads, which provide fiber, minerals and the B and E vitamin complexes. Most bread you find today is made by mass production methods using ingredients like hydrogenated vegetable oils, monoacetyltartaric acid, disodium dihydrogen diphosphate, and other artificial chemicals.

13. Avoid constipation - eat plenty of raw fruits and vegetables and drink plenty of water during the day. Supplement with a whole food based gastrointestinal purification product.

14. Avoid excessive saturated or hydrogenated fats and incorporate essential fatty acid oil blends into your diet as a replacement. Recommended oils include cold pressed organic hemp seed oil, flax seed oil, and Essential Oil Balance by Omega.

15. Help someone out, no matter how small or grand the task, each day.

16. Smile…Laugh

23.2 Exercise

Exercise plays a critical role in the purification process. Exercise is a life-long commitment that, if practiced with gratitude for the ability to move around and sweat, will offer a great return on one's investment of time and energy. Exercise aids in excreting toxins and restoring systemic balance. It also helps to maintain or increase bone and muscle mass, as well as strength and endurance. Beginning an exercise program that entails sweating for at least 20 minutes, five times per week, will have a positive impact on the entire process. Before and after a purification program, aerobic activities like running, walking, cycling, skiing, rock-climbing and swimming are all good options for working up a sweat. During a purification program, particularly a 21-day program, gentle to moderate exercises such as yoga, chi kung and tai chi are ideal. These exercises will support the process by restoring vitality, storing physical energy which may decrease initially as one's caloric intake is restricted, massaging organs in the abdominal cavity, stimulating blood circulation, improving strength, flexibility and balance and encouraging mental relaxation-all ideal states to be in during a purification process. Below are some of the primary benefits of aerobic exercise on the body, validated by research studies.

Scientifically validated effects of exercise on the body

- Stimulates the release of toxins and waste materials from cells[21,24]
- Improves circulation[4,9,38]
- Improves lipid profile[20,29]
- Improves fertility[10]
- Maintains healthy cardiovascular function[7,13,17,26]
- Aids in weight reduction[36]
- Increases body temperature[19]
- Maintains healthy blood sugar levels[6]
- Restores healthy lung function[1,34,37]
- Increases flexibility and strength[3,27,30]
- Improves bone structure[8,27,30]
- Improves mental outlook[22,31]

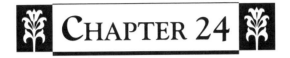

CHAPTER 24

MANUAL LYMPHATIC DRAINAGE

"To array a man's will against his sickness is the supreme art of medicine."
—Beecher

24

Manual Lymphatic Drainage

Manual lymphatic drainage (MLD) is a valid adjunctive method of treatment for lymphedema and toxicity. Developed by Emil and Estrid Vodder in Denmark in the 1930's, this body work technique has proven its effectiveness in increasing the flow of lymph in the interstitial spaces thereby delivering essential nutrients to cells and facilitating the release of stored toxins.[2,5,16,23] This type of body work mechanically displaces lymph through gaps between endothelial cells of the collecting lymph vessels.

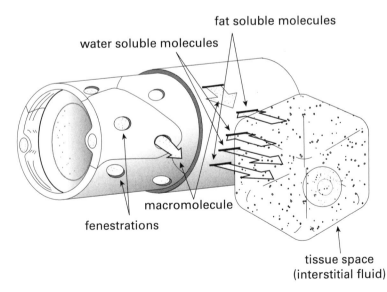

Figure 24.1
Capillary showing gaps (fenestrations) between endothelial cells through which lymph is displaced by MLD.

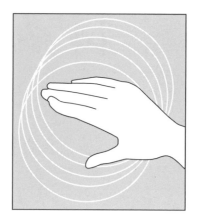

Figure 24.2
Circular hand motions are used in Manual Lymphatic Technique

The actual technique includes various circular finger pressure motions covering small sections of the skin, as well as circular hand motions covering larger areas of the skin.

Manual lymphatic drainage should only be practiced by a healthcare professional specifically trained in this method of large-surface massage. The basic principles of MLD are:

• The skin should always be kneaded and never stroked.

• The proximal area (area closer to the center of the body) is treated first, followed by treatment of the distal parts of the body. This method allows room for fluid that has naturally accumulated in the distal portions of the body to flow towards the proximal areas of the body.

• The techniques and derivations thereof are repeated rhythmically, usually five to seven times, either localized to an area working in stationary circles or in expanding spirals.

• The skin should never redden

• This technique should never elicit pain

This technique by Vodder must be executed precisely, as the more exacting the technique, the more demonstrable the results, particularly on a patient that is actively participating in a clinical purification program. Some contraindications to note when administering any type of body work are:

- fever

- external injury to the skin

- inflammation

- high blood pressure

- recent consumption of nicotine or alcohol

- full stomach

- concussion

- sprain

- unmended broken bone

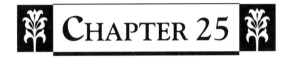

CHAPTER 25

YOGA AND BREATHING

"Yoga is not about learning to stand on your head,
it is about learning to stand on your own two feet."
—Cintra

25

>>>)(<<<

YOGA AND BREATHING

T he word "yoga" is derived from the verbal root, yuj, meaning to yoke or harness. Yoga is the process of unifying one's mind body and soul in order to express the energy of one's true nature. In the author's professional opinion, based on personal experience with practicing and teaching yoga, hatha yoga (a type of yoga referred to as "physical" yoga) is the ideal exercise practice while going through a clinical purification program. *Just as one uses alchemic principles to create a purification formula from herbs and foods to address the functioning of specific organs in the body, hatha yoga involves the alchemic reprogramming of mind and body that serves to release toxins and purify the soul.*

The word "hatha" is derived from the Sanskrit root, ha (sun) and tha (moon), and is the equalization and stabilization of the sun-moon (yin-yang) life-force. The purpose of Hatha yoga is to free the body and mind from dysfunctional blockages. With respect to the Clinical Purification™ Process, this equates to the elimination of exogenous and endogenous toxins. Hatha yoga involves a methodical and integrative approach to stretching and contracting different muscle groups to strengthen and lengthen opposing muscles. Hatha also re-aligns the skeleton and applies weight to vital bones to maintain and increase bone density. At the same time and perhaps less obviously, Hatha yoga also gently massages all internal organs.

Following is a series of basic yoga postures that one can begin practicing at home. It is important to be in a warm room, with comfortable clothes and preferably barefoot. When practicing these postures, one must be mindful of his/her body, backing off when one feels pain and slowly extending beyond the point of resistance only when one feels ready to do so. Those who practice yoga regularly often notice a gradual increase in strength, flexibility and balance. *The most critical factor when practicing yoga is to be mindful of one's breath.*[3,26,31,34,37]

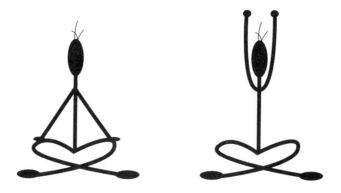

Sit / Easy Position - Sukhasana

A starting position that helps focus awareness on breathing and the body; helps strengthen lower back and open the groin and hips.

Sit cross-legged with hands on knees. Focus on your breath. Keep your spine straight and push the sit bones down into the floor. Allow the knees to gently lower. If the knees rise above your hips, sit on a cushion or block. This will help support your back and hips. Take 5-10 slow, deep breaths. On the next inhale, raise your arms over your head. Exhale and bring your arms down slowly. Repeat 5-7 times.

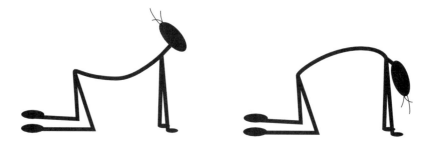

Dog and Cat

Increases flexibility of the spine.

Begin on your hands and knees. Keep your hands just in front of your shoulders, your legs about hip width apart. As you inhale, tilt the tailbone and pelvis up, and let the spine curve downward, dropping the stomach low, and lift your head up. Stretch gently. As you exhale, move into cat by reversing the spinal bend, tilting the pelvis down, drawing the spine up and pulling the chest and stomach in. Repeat several times, flowing smoothly from dog into cat, and cat back into dog.

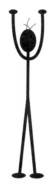

Mountain - Tadasana

Improves posture, balance and self-awareness.

Stand with feet together, hands at your sides, eyes looking forward. Raise your toes, fan them open, then place them back down on the floor. Feel your heel, outside of your foot, toes and ball of your foot all in contact with the floor. Tilt your pubic bone slightly forward. Raise your chest up and out, but within reason - this isn't the army and you're not standing at attention. Raise your head up and lengthen the neck by lifting the base of your skull toward the ceiling. Stretch the pinky on each hand downward, then balance that movement by stretching your index fingers. Push into the floor with your feet and raise your legs, first the calves and then the thighs.

Breathe. Hold the posture, but try not to tense up. Breathe. As you inhale, imagine the breath coming up through the floor, rising through your legs and torso and up into your head. Reverse the process on the exhale and watch your breath as it passes down from your head, through your chest and stomach, legs and feet.

Hold for 5 to 10 breaths, relax and repeat.

On your next inhale, raise your arms over head (Urdhava Hastasana) and hold for several breaths. Lower your arms on an exhale.

As a warm up, try synchronizing the raising and lowering of your arms with your breath - raise, inhale; lower, exhale. Repeat 5 times.

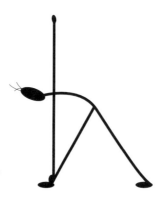

Forward Bend or Extension - Uttanasana II

Stretches the legs and spine, rests the heart and neck, relaxes mind and body

Begin standing straight in Mountain pose or Tadasana. Inhale and raise the arms overhead. Exhale, bend at the hips, bring the arms forward and down until you touch the floor. It's okay to bend your knees, especially if you're feeling stiff. Either grasp your ankles or just leave your hands on the floor and breathe several times. Repeat 3-5 times. On your last bend, hold the position for 5 or 10 breaths. To come out of the pose, curl upward as if pulling yourself up one vertebrae at a time, stacking one on top of another, and leaving the head hanging down until last.

Trikonasana - the Triangle

Stretches the spine, opens the torso, improves balance and concentration.

Start with your legs spread 3-4 feet apart, feet parallel. Turn your left foot 90 degrees to the left and your right foot about 45 degrees inward. Inhale and raise both arms so they're parallel with the floor. Exhale, turn your head to the left and look down your left arm toward your outstretched fingers. Check that your left knee is aligned with your left ankle. Take a deep breath and stretch outward to the left, tilting the left hip down and the right hip up. When you've stretched as far as you can, pivot your arms, letting your left hand reach down and come to rest against the inside of your calf, while your right arms points straight up. Turn and look up at your right hand. Breathe deeply for several breaths. Inhale, and straighten up. Exhale, lower your arms. Put your hands on your hips and pivot on your heels, bringing your feet to face front. Repeat the posture on the other side.

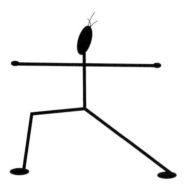

Warrior I I - Virabhadrasana II

Strengthens legs and arms; improves balance and concentration; builds confidence.

Begin in mountain pose with feet together and hands at side. Place your feet 4-5 feet apart. Turn your right foot about 45 degrees to the left. Turn your left foot 90 degrees to the left so that it is pointing straight out to the side. Slowly bend the left knee until the thigh is parallel with the floor, but keep the knee either behind or directly over your ankle. Raise your arms overhead. Then slowly lower them until your left arm is pointing straight ahead and your right arm is pointing back. Concentrate on a spot in front of you and breathe. Take 4 or 5 deep breaths, lower your arms, bring your legs together. Reverse the position.

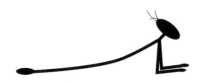

The Cobra - Bhujangasana

Stretches the spine, strengthens the back and arms, opens the chest and heart.

Lay down on your stomach. Keep your legs together, arms at your side, close to your body, with your hands by your chest.

Step 1: Inhaling, slowly raise your head and chest as high as it will go. Keep your buttocks muscles tight to protect your lower back. Keep your head up and chest. Breathe several times and then come down. Repeat as necessary.

Step 2: Follow the steps above. When you've gone as high as you can, gently raise your hands off of the floor stretching the spine even more. Only go as far as you are comfortable. Your pelvis should always remain on the floor. Breathe several times and come down.

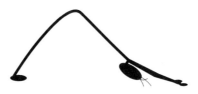

Downward Facing Dog - Adho Mukha Svanasana

Builds strength, flexibility and awareness; stretches the spine and hamstrings; rests the heart.

Start on your hands and knees. Keep your legs about hip width apart and your arms shoulder width apart. Your middle fingers should be parallel, pointing straight ahead. Roll your elbows so that the eye or inner elbow is facing forward. Inhale and curl your toes under, as if getting ready to stand on your toes. Exhale and straighten your legs; push upward with your arms. The goal is to lengthen the spine while keeping your legs straight and your feet flat on the ground. However, in the beginning it's okay to bend the knees a bit and to keep your heels raised. The important thing is to work on lengthening the spine. Don't let your shoulders creep up by your ears -- keep them down. Weight should be evenly distributed between your hands and feet. Hold the position for a few breaths. Come down on and exhale. Repeat several times, synchronizing with your breath: up on the exhale and down on the inhale.

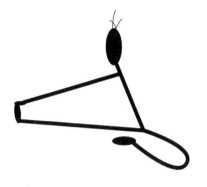

Head to Knee - Janu Shirshasana

Stretches and opens back and hamstrings, improves flexibility

Sit on the floor with legs extended in front of you. Bend one leg, bringing the heel of the foot as close to the groin as possible. You may want to place a pillow under the bent knee for comfort. Make sure your sitz bones are firmly grounded on the floor and that your spine is straight. Turn your body slightly so you face out over the extended leg. Inhale and raise your arms over head. Exhale and begin to move forward slowly. Try to keep the back as straight as possible. Instead of bending at the hips, focus on lifting the tailbone and rolling forward on your sitz bones. Inhale and lengthen and straighten the spine. Exhale and roll forward, however slightly. To get a bit more forward movement, engage your quadriceps (thigh muscles) as you move forward. This releases the hamstrings, giving you a bit more flexibility. When you've moved as far forward as you can, lower the arms and grasp your foot, or leg. Hold the position for a moment and breathe. Then on the next exhale gently pull yourself forward. Go slowly and remember to keep the back straight. When done, straighten up and do the other side.

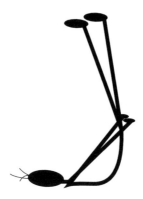

Half Shoulderstand - Ardha Sarvangasana

Promotes proper thyroid function, strengthens abdomen, stretches upper back, improves blood circulation, induces relaxation

You probably remember doing this as a kid. Lie on your back and lift your legs up into air. Place your hands on your lower back for support, resting your elbows and lower arms on the ground. Make sure your weight is on your shoulders and mid to upper back -- not your neck. Breathe deeply and hold the posture for at least 5-10 breaths, increasing the hold over time. To come down, slowly lower your legs, keeping them very straight - a little workout for your abdominal muscles.

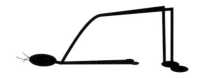

The Bridge - Sethu Bandhasa

Increases flexibility and suppleness; strengthens the lower back and abdominal muscles; opens the chest.

Lay on your back with your knees up and hands at your side Your feet should be near your buttocks about six inches apart. To begin, gently raise and lower your tail. Then, slowly, raise the tailbone and continue lifting the spine, trying to move one vertebra at a time until your entire back is arched upward. Push firmly with your feet. Keep your knees straight and close together. Breathe deeply into your chest. Clasp your hands under your back and push against the floor.

Take five slow, deep breaths.

Come down slowly and repeat.

The Corpse - Savasana

Relaxes and refreshes the body and mind, relieves stress and anxiety, quiets the mind

Possibly the most important posture, the Corpse, is as deceptively simple as Tadasana, the Mountain pose. Usually performed at the end of a session, the goal is conscious relaxation. Many people find the "conscious" part the most difficult because it is very easy to drift off to sleep while doing Savasana. Begin by lying on your back, feet slightly apart, arms at your sides with palms facing up. Close your eyes and take several slow, deep breaths. Allow your body to sink into the ground. Try focusing on a specific part of the body and willing it to relax. For example, start with your feet, imagine the muscles and skin relaxing, letting go and slowly melting into the floor. From your feet, move on to your calves, thighs and so on up to your face and head. Then simply breathe and relax. Stay in the pose for at least 5-10 minutes.

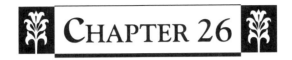

CHAPTER 26

SAUNA THERAPY

"Give me the power to create a fever, and I shall cure any disease."
– Hippocrates

26

SAUNA THERAPY

Sauna therapy is a thermal therapy that has been recognized throughout history as a viable means of relaxing and cleansing the body, improving overall health, and promoting a sense of well-being. From Finland to India to North America, saunas are recommended by medical professionals as a safe and effective adjunctive therapy for detoxification. It is a practical means of stimulating the release of non-essential or toxic trace metals such as nickel, cadmium, and lead through sweat. The therapeutic rationale for using sauna therapy is that overheating the body, and hence inducing an artificial fever, stimulates metabolism, inhibits the growth of bacteria, increases the ability of all vital organs, and increases the capacity of the skin to eliminate, detoxify and cleanse via profuse sweating.

A sauna is a relatively airtight, though ventilated, room usually made of poplar, glass, tile, concrete or wood. There are two major types of saunas, wet or steam saunas, and dry saunas. In both cases, the temperature should remain between 140 and 170 degrees Fahrenheit. Ideally, a patient will begin by remaining in a sauna for 15 minutes, followed by a cold shower, then repeat the process for approximately one hour. As one becomes acclimated to the therapy, he or she can gradually increase the time of this cycle to 2 hours per day. It is important that the patient remains hydrated throughout the process.

26.1 Safety of Sauna Therapy

Sauna therapy is generally well tolerated by most healthy adults and children. This therapy has been shown to cause transient changes in hormones and cardiovascular function. However, sauna therapy does not influence fertility and it is considered a safe treatment during uncomplicated pregnancies in healthy women.[11] With regard to cardiovascular health, recent research shows that repeated sauna therapy upregulates endothelial nitro oxide synthase expression in arterial endothelium thereby improving the hemodynamics, endothelial function and clinical symptoms in patients with chronic heart failure.[14] Further, some studies suggest that long-term sauna therapy may improve the left ventricular ejection fraction in patients with chronic congestive heart failure, and it may help lower blood pressure in hypertensive patients.[11,18] Patients with chronic bronchitis and asthma may benefit from the transient improvements in pulmonary function that occur because of sauna therapy. Further, patients with rheumatic disease can safely employ sauna therapy as a means of improving joint mobility and relieving pain.[11]

26.2 Contraindications

Contraindications to sauna therapy include:

• Recent Myocardial Infarction

• Unstable Angina Pectoris

• Severe Aortic Stenosis

• Alcoholism or recent alcohol consumption

• Heart Disease

• Kidney Disease

• Anemia

• Pregnant Women should be monitored closely by a qualified healthcare professional

26.3 Overview

Sauna therapy is an excellent complimentary modality to employ with the process of Clinical Purification.™

In summary, the major benefits of sauna therapy include[11,14,18,28,32] :

• Release of accumulated toxins such as pesticides, PCBs, drug residues, acidic wastes and non-essential trace metals

• Improvement in symptoms of Atopic Dermatitis

• Increased oxygenation of the tissues and cells

• Increased circulation, oxygen and nutrient delivery within the body

• Improvement in immune function

• Improved cardiovascular function

• Improved pulmonary function

• Alleviation of pain and improved joint mobility

• Improved psoriatic conditions

• Relief of symptoms of asthma and chronic bronchitis

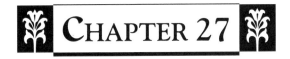

CHAPTER 27

DRY SKIN BRUSHING

"Healing is a matter of time, but it is sometimes also a matter of opportunity."
— Hippocrates

27

Dry Skin Brushing

As the largest eliminative organ, the skin plays a vital role in ridding the body of toxins. As part of the Clinical Purification™ process, healthcare practitioners can recommend dry skin brushing to their patients to open up the pores of the skin and support lymphatic cleansing. When the pores are not clogged with dead cells and the lymphatic system is cleansed, the body is able to carry out the function of eliminating toxins and waste material.[12]

27.1 How to Skin Brush

It is important to practice dry skin brushing every day during the Clinical Purification™ process. The best time to dry skin brush is upon rising, prior to showering, when the skin is completely dry. The brush, which must be completely dry, is a natural vegetable-bristle brush with a long handle to aid in brushing hard- to- reach areas of the body. Begin by gently brushing with one-stroke movements. If the skin reddens, the patient is brushing too hard. The basic principle is to brush from the outermost points of one's body (hands and feet) towards the center. Start by brushing from the feet to the abdomen, then from the hands up to the arms towards the heart. Brush across the upper back and down the front and back of the torso. One should aim to cover the entire surface of the skin.[12] The process takes between three and five minutes to complete.

27.2 Overview

Dry skin brushing is a useful adjunctive therapy that helps to release toxins from the body.

Additionally, the process of dry skin brushing:

• Boosts immune function

• Stimulates the lymphatic system

• Stimulates the circulatory system.[35]

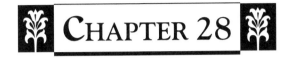

CHAPTER 28

CONSTITUTIONAL HYDROTHERAPY

"In one drop of water are found all the secrets of all the oceans."
–Gibran

28

CONSTITUTIONAL HYDROTHERAPY

ydrotherapy is a treatment modality that employs water, "hydro" to treat disease, "therapy." The treatment makes use of the body's response to hot and cold applications. The body's initial reaction to cold is stimulation, with a secondary reaction of invigoration and tonification. This secondary reaction results in perspiration and a slowed pulse rate. The body's primary response to a heat application is stimulation with a secondary depressive or sedative reaction. This secondary reaction causes an increased pulse rate, a decrease in perspiration and muscular weakness. Water therapy is an ideal modality to use during the Clinical Purification™ process as it successfully increases circulation of the blood and lymph, thereby cleansing the skin and ridding the body of toxic waste.

28.1 History of Hydrotherapy

cornerstone of naturopathic medicine, the practice of Hydrotherapy, has stood the test of time as a priceless and ageless treatment modality. Beginning in the late 1600's in England, **Dr. John Floyer (1649-1734)** advocated the use of cold baths in his book, *The History of Hot and Cold Bathing*. This book influenced **Dr. Johann Hahn (1696-1773)** who was influential in establishing the principles of modern hydrotherapy in Germany.

Johann Hahn together with his father and brother, also physicians, influenced **Vincent Priessnitz (1799-1852)**, a lay practitioner, who was actually introduced to the therapy by an elderly neighbor who used water to treat his cattle's bruises and tumors. By 1830, Priessnitz was so successful with treating acquaintances with water that the Austrian government awarded him special authority to treat patients with his therapeutic methods.

Father Sebastian Kneipp (1821-1897) followed Priessnitz in his pursuit of popularizing hydrotherapy, later becoming one of the world's most famous water cure doctors, also having a very strong and direct influence on the field of Naturopathic Medicine* in the United States. Curing

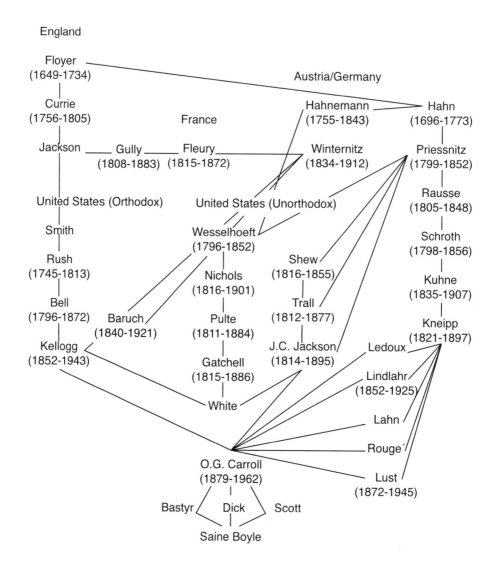

Figure 28.1
Direct and indirect connections between key hydrotherapy practitioners.[33]

himself from tuberculosis by repeated immersions in the Danube River, Kneipp rose to international prominence and became known as the "cholera vicar" because of the many lives he saved with his water cure during an epidemic. He wrote 22 books and cured thousands, rarely charging a fee and using gifts from patients to set up sanitariums.

Benedict Lust (1872-1943) was introduced to the field by Kneipp who cured Lust of tuberculosis. Kneipp commissioned Lust to introduce his work to the United States which Lust gratefully proceeded to do, founding, in 1896, the American Naturopathic Association*.

Another successful water cure practitioner of the late 1800's was **John Harvey Kellogg (1852-1943)** who helped to set up a sanitarium in Michigan, the Battle Creek Sanitarium, where he employed water treatments and conducted numerous comparative experiments on the different water treatments he used. In 1901 Kellogg wrote a definitive text on hydrotherapy entitled, "Rational Hydrotherapy," considered a classic work by Naturopathic Doctors throughout the world.

Dr. O.G. Carroll (1879-1962) is the father of Constitutional Hydrotherapy. While the term hydrotherapy represents all modalities that employ water as the primary tool, constitutional hydrotherapy is a very specific method of hydrotherapy that was defined and perfected by Dr. Carroll. Trained as a chiropractor from Cleveland Chiropractic College in Chicago at the time, he later moved to Spokane Washington and, in 1908, became one of the first naturopathic practitioners in the west. He was infamous for curing the most challenging of cases, and at one point curing Dr. Kellogg's wife of asthma. **Dr. John Bastyr,** considered one of the greatest naturopaths of our time, studied closely with Dr. Carroll. Numerous other practitioners were and are influential in popularizing the use of hydrotherapy as a primary treatment modality. Following is a flow chart that shows the direct and indirect influential relationships between all major water cure practitioners.

* The Principles of Naturopathic Medicine are outlined within the Naturopathic Physician's Oath, which can be found in Appendix H. Naturopathic Doctors (N.D.'s or N.M.D.'s) are general primary care practitioners trained as specialists in natural medicine. They are educated in the conventional medical sciences, but they are not orthodox medical doctors (M.D.'s). Naturopathic doctors restore health using therapies from the sciences of clinical purification or detoxification, clinical nutrition, herbal medicine, homeopathy, counseling, acupuncture, and manipulation. They tailor these approaches to the needs of the individual patient or client. Naturopathic therapies are effective in treating most health problems, whether acute or chronic. Naturopathic doctors cooperate with all other branches of medical sciences, referring clients to other practitioners for diagnosis or treatment when appropriate. Naturopathic Doctors that qualify for licensure in their state of practice hold a Doctor of Naturopathic Medicine degree from a four-year graduate level naturopathic medical college. For more information about naturopathic medicine in the United States, and reputable naturopathic medical colleges, contact the American Association of Naturopathic Physicians at www.naturopathic.org.

28.2 Constitutional Hydrotherapy

Constitutional hydrotherapy is a complex water treatment that requires the skill of a highly trained therapist. Appendix D offers guidelines to the patient and practitioner for trying a modified version of constitutional hydrotherapy. However, the author does not recommend blind adherence to the protocol, as the clinical judgment of a trained practitioner in this treatment modality will produce results that are far more effectual. Dr. Andre Saine, N.D. and Dr. Wayne Boyle, N.D.'s book, *Lectures in Naturopathic Hydrotherapy* is recommended for practitioners interested in utilizing this therapy.

28.3 Primary Indications for Use

- Clinical Purification™

- Arthritis

- Circulatory challenges

- Depression

- Diabetes

- Digestive disturbances

- Eczema

- Female reproductive health

- Immunodeficiency conditions

- Infectious diseases

- Obesity

- Psoriasis

- Respiratory challenges

28.4 Contraindications

- Acute asthma

- Acute bladder infection

- Anemia

- Fear of therapy

- Malignant fever

- Oral temperature under 97 degrees Fahrenheit

28.5 Modified Constitutional Hydrotherapy Guidelines

This modified Constitutional Hydrotherapy technique involves a series of hot and cold compress applications to the chest, abdomen and back.

Materials:

Two 100% wool blankets
One pillow
Massage or treatment table (preferable but not required)
Four bath-sized towels
Sink or bucket filled with ice cubes and cold water
Sink or bucket filled with hot water

Guidelines for Treatment:

1. Place one wool blanket length wise along the treatment table with one pillow at head of table.

2. Instruct patient to undress from the waist up, lie face up on the table and cover him/herself with the other blanket.

3. Soak two towels in hot water and wring enough so that they do not drip. Test the towels on the wrist to assure that they do not burn the patient.

4. Expose the patient's chest and abdomen and place the hot towels, one directly upon the other, slowly, over the chest and abdomen. Cover the patient immediately with the blanket and wait 5 minutes.

5. During that time, prepare one cold towel by soaking it in an ice water bath and gently ring out so that it does not drip, and prepare one hot towel as done previously.

6. After 5 minutes, open the patient's blanket and place the new hot towel upon the two towels that are already there. Quickly flip all three towels over so that the new hot towel is now on the patient's skin. Remove the other two towels.

7. Immediately place the cold towel over the new hot towel and again flip both towels so that the cold towel is now touching the patient.

8. Quickly remove the hot towel and cover the patient completely with the blanket.

9. Wait ten minutes and then check to see if the patient has warmed the previously cold towel. If not, wait another 3 minutes and re-check. If the towel is warm, remove it and have the patient turn over, face down. If the towel fails to warm, repeat until the patient is able to warm the towel.

10. Repeat the entire process on the backside.

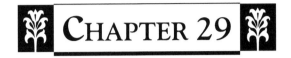

CHAPTER 29

COLONIC THERAPY / ENEMAS

"Prevention is better than cure."
—Erasmus

29

COLONIC THERAPY / ENEMAS

Healthcare practitioners throughout history have advocated the use of enemas as a means of cleansing the body and improving health. In 1917, Dr. Kellogg reported in the Journal of American Medicine that "in more than 40,000 cases, as a result of diet, exercises and enema, (in all but twenty cases), [Dr. Kellogg] had used no surgery for the treatment of gastrointestinal disease in his patients." As a Naturopathic Physician, the author has consistently seen the benefits of enemas for maintenance and restoration of health, particularly when recommend as part of a clinical purification program.[25,39,40]

One might consider the age-old saying, "sickness and health begin in the colon" when evaluating the benefits of colonic therapy during a Clinical Purification™ program. When a patient chooses to begin a Clinical Purification™ protocol, it is critical that their colon is functioning optimally, as the majority of toxins pulled out of storage by detoxifying herbs and nutrient complexes must be eliminated via the colon. If the colon is not functioning well, these toxins can be re-circulated through the system causing autointoxication, which may very well be the origin of most symptoms of a so-called "healing crisis." Dr. Bernard Jensen, D.C., warned that "when toxins are being assimilated or created in the body faster than they can be gotten rid of, or when one or more of the eliminative systems are under active, trouble lies ahead. I am convinced that toxic accumulations in the body create the necessary preconditions for disease to develop."[15]

29.1 Directions for Administering an Enema

Enema bags or colema boards are useful tools for cleansing your colon at home. The enema bag is cheaper than a colema board, holds much less water (thus less water gets into the colon), and is not done over the toilet, whereas a colema board is done over the toilet.

Hang the enema bag at least 18 inches above your body. Before you fill the bag, make sure the tubing clamp is shut tight so that the content of the bag does not leak out. Fill the bag with warm (comfortable to touch), purified, distilled or reverse osmosis water. Lubricate the rectal tip with a non-petroleum lubricant like vitamin E. Lie on your back on a towel on the floor, or even in a tepid water bath and insert the rectal tip. Open the tubing clamp. Let as much liquid into your colon as you feel comfortable with and then re-clamp the tubing. At this point, either massage your colon from left to right, descending colon to ascending colon, in small circular motions or lift your buttocks off the ground with your legs to further move the liquid into your colon. Try to retain the enema for about 15 minutes or longer. Evacuate whenever you need to.

Make sure you haven't ingested anything for 2 hours prior to starting the enema. After you complete your enema, wait at least 45 minutes before ingesting anything.

Colema Boards are more expensive, hold 4-5 gallons of water and are done over the toilet. You fill the bucket with room temperature, reverse osmosis water. It must sit one to two feet above your body. You will have to get suction in the hose before it will flow down. To do this, fill the plastic hose up with water and let some of it out. This will create suction. Clamp the tube and put one end in the bucket.

One end of the colema board lies over the toilet bowl and the other end lies on a chair. Place one or two towels on the board for comfort. Lubricate the plastic tubing which goes into the rectum. Lie down and insert the tube into the rectum. Allow the water to follow into your colon. At first, do not try to hold too much water. If you feel any pressure, then simply "let go" and the water will come pouring out into the toilet. The more you get used to taking home colonics, the more you will know exactly how much you can hold.

Some people feel much more at ease having a trained professional assisting them to clean their colon. When that is the case, consider going to a colon hydrotherapist for a professional colonic treatment.

29.2 Enema Recipe

Olive Oil/Aloe Vera: In an enema bag, pour one cup of organic olive oil and one cup of organic aloe vera juice. Open four whole food-based fiber capsules and mix with liquid. Slowly pour into colon with enema bag. Hold as long as you are able. This will soothe the intestinal lining during inflammation as well as clean the colon.

PART 3
CLINICAL REFERENCES

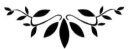

(CHAPTERS 23-29)

1.   Behera, D. 1998. Yoga therapy in chronic bronchitis. *J Assoc Physicians India* 46(2): 207-208.
2.   Casley-Smith, J. R. et al. 1998. Treatment for lymphedema of the arm--the Casley-Smith method: A noninvasive method produces continued reduction. *Cancer* 83(12 Suppl American): 2843-2860.
3.   Corliss, R. 2001. The power of yoga. *Time* 157(16): 54-62.
4.   Dornyei, G. et al. 2000. Regular exercise enhances blood pressure lowering effect of acetylcholine by increased contribution of nitric oxide. *Acta Physiol Hung* 87(2): 127-138.
5.   Evrard-Bras, M. et al. 2000. Manual lymphatic drainage. *Rev Prat* 50(11): 1199-1203.
6.   Fritz, T. and U. Rosenqvist. 2001. Walking for exercise - immediate effect on blood glucose levels in type 2 diabetes. *Scand J Prim Health Care* 19(1): 31-33.
7.   Georgiou, D. et al. 2001. Cost-effectiveness analysis of long-term moderate exercise training in chronic heart failure. *Am J Cardiol* 87(8): 984-988; A4.
8.   Gustavsson, A. et al. 2000. Osteocalcin gene polymorphism is related to bone density in healthy adolescent females. *Osteoporos Int* 11(10): 847-851.
9.   Gustafsson, T. and C. J. Sundberg. 2000. Expression of angiogenic growth factors in human skeletal muscle in response to a singular bout of exercise. *Am J Physiol Heart Circ Physiol* 279(6): H3144-H3145.
10.   Hally, S. S. 1998. Nutrition in reproductive health. *J Nurse Midwifery* 43(6): 459-470.
11.   Hannuksela, M. L. and S. Ellahham. 2001. Benefits and risks of sauna bathing. *Am J Med* 110(2): 118-126.
12.   Henke, F. 2000. Alternative skin care: Fit and revitalized with the aid of dry brushing. *Pflege Z* 53(2): 95-96.
13.   Hoyt, R. E. and L. S. Bowling. 2001. Reducing readmissions for congestive heart failure. *Am Fam Physician* 63(8): 1593-1598.
14.   Ikeda, Y. et al. 2001. Repeated thermal therapy upregulates arterial endothelial nitric oxide synthase expression in Syrian golden hamsters. *Jpn Circ J* 65(5): 434-438.
15.   Jensen, B. 1981. Tissue Cleansing Through Bowel Manangement. Bernard Jensen International.
16.   Kasseroller, R. G. 1998. The Vodder School: The Vodder method. *Cancer* 83(12 Suppl American): 2840-2842.
17.   Kavanagh, T. 2001. Exercise in the primary prevention of coronary artery disease. *Can J Cardiol* 17(2): 155-161.
18.   Keast, M. L. and K. B. Adamo. 2000. The Finnish sauna bath and its use in patients with cardiovascular disease. *J Cardiopulm Rehabil* 20(4): 225-230.
19.   Kenny, G. P. et al. 1999. The effect of dynamic exercise on resting cold thermoregulatory responses measured during water immersion. *Eur J Appl Physiol Occup Physiol* 79(6): 495-499.
20.   Kim, J. R. et al. 2001. Effect of exercise intensity and frequency on lipid levels in men with coronary heart disease: Training Level Comparison Trial. *Am J Cardiol* 87(8): 942-946; A3.
21.   Kilburn, K. H. et al. 1989. Neurobehavioral dysfunction in firemen exposed to polycholorinated biphenyls (PCBs): Possible improvement after detoxification. *Arch Environ Health* 44(6): 345-350. Comment in *Arch Environ Health*, 1991 Jul-Aug; 46(4): 254-255.
22.   Lawlor, D. A. and S. W. Hopker. 2001. The effectiveness of exercise as an intervention in the management of depression: Systematic review and meta-regression analysis of randomised controlled trials. *BMJ* 322(7289): 763-767.
23.   Leduc, O. et al. 1998. The physical treatment of upper limb edema. *Cancer* 83(12 Suppl American): 2835-2839.
24.   Lew, H. and A. Quintanilha. 1991. Effects of endurance training and exercise on tissue antioxidative capacity and acetaminophen detoxification. *Eur J Drug Metab Pharmacokinet* 16(1): 59-68.
25.   Lipski, E. 2000. Digestive Wellness. Keats Publishing.
26.   Manchanda, S. C. et al. 2000. Retardation of coronary atherosclerosis with yoga lifestyle intervention. *J Assoc Physicians India* 48(7): 687-694.
27.   Notomi , T. et al. 2000. A comparison of resistance and aerobic training for mass, strength and turnover of bone in growing rats. *Eur J Appl Physiol* 83(6): 469-474.
28.   Pashkov, V. K. et al. 2000. The sauna in the treatment of children with atopic dermatitis. *Vopr Kurortol Fizioter Lech Fiz Kult* (4):37-39.
29.   Pignone, M. P. et al. 2001. Screening and treating adults for lipid disorders. *Am J Prev Med* 20(3 Suppl): 77-89.
30.   Proctor, D. N. et al. 2000. Relative influence of physical activity, muscle mass and strength on bone density. *Osteoporos Int* 11(11): 944-952.
31.   Ray, U. S. et al. 2001. Effect of yogic exercises on physical and mental health of young fellowship course trainees. *Indian J Physiol Pharmacol* 45(1): 37-53.
32.   Saikhun, J. et al. 1998. Effects of sauna on sperm movement characteristics of normal men measured by computer-assisted sperm analysis. *Int J Androl* 21(6): 358-363.
33.   Saine, A. and W. Boyle. 1988. Lectures in Naturopathic Hydrotherapy. East Palestine, OH: Buckeye Naturopathic Press.

34. Sathyaprabha, T. N. et al. 2001. Efficacy of naturopathy and yoga in bronchial asthma--a self controlled matched scientific study. *Indian J Physiol Pharmacol* 45(1): 80-86.
35. Soltanoff, J. 1988. Natural Healing. Washington, D.C.: Warner Books.
36. Stromme, S. B. and A. T. Hostmark. 2000. Physical activity, overweight and obesity. *Tidsskr Nor Laegeforen* 120(29): 3578-3582.
37. Telles, S. et al. 2000. Oxygen consumption and respiration following two yoga relaxation techniques. *Appl Psychophysiol Biofeedback* 25(4): 221-227.
38. Vissing, J. 2000. Muscle reflex and central motor control of neuroendocrine activity, glucose homeostasis and circulation during exercise. *Acta Physiol Scand Suppl* 647: 1-26.
39. Watson, B. 1999. Notes from a lecture at a International Association of Colon Hydrotherapy Convention, 1999.
40. Weil, A. 1998. Health and Healing. Houghton Mifflin Company.

PART 4

CLINICAL PURIFICATION PROTOCOLS

"There is in all visible things… a hidden wholeness."
—Thomas Merton

CLINICAL PURIFICATION PROTOCOLS

INTRODUCTION

Following this introduction are three separate 21 day programs, based on the research outlined in this book, that will effectively carry practitioners and their patients through the Clinical Purification™ process. The details of each program are all written in a "patient handout" format so that the practitioner has a tool that he or she may use to easily explain the process to the patient or client. As all practitioners realize at some point in their career, every patient that comes through the door is in a different place; physically, mentally, emotionally and spiritually. The protocols that follow represent the "scientific" tools needed for carrying out the Clinical Purification™ process. The practitioner must employ whatever "artistic" tool necessary to determine which program is best suited for the individual patient to assure compliance and a positive outcome. The art of practicing medicine is just as crucial as the science of medicine when it comes to addressing health and disease through Clinical Purification.™

Program One ~ Intensity Level Mild

Program One is the least complicated of the three programs and will most likely render the most patient compliance. The program involves the principle of caloric restriction without malnutrition. Patients will cut all meal portions in half for a period of 21 days, drink meal replacement shakes before at least one meal per day, and follow a whole food and herb-based supplement program that addresses all organs that affect the purification process. For the first 7 days (week one) the patient will utilize a systemic cleansing product from a high quality supplement manufacturer that includes the whole food and herbal ingredients outlined in this book. For the next 14 days (weeks two and three) the patient will take a gastrointestinal/fiber product that includes psyllium, apple pectin, and fenugreek seeds to maintain optimal gastrointestinal function during the process.

Program Two ~ Intensity Level Moderate

Program Two is more involved and restrictive, although the end result is especially profound. Nothing worth having is ever easy. The patient is guided to remove select foods from the diet for a period of 21 days. The patient is encouraged to mindfully address mental, emotional and spiritual issues that may come up in the process. Additionally, it is important for the patient and practitioner to address the need for utilizing complimentary methods of purification such as colon irrigation, systemic hydrotherapy, lymphatic massage and skin brushing. The supplement and meal replacement recommendations are identical to Program One.

Program Three ~ Intensity Level Optimal

Program Three will yield the most profound results of the three. The first 7 days (week one) eliminates all foods and drinks from the diet except for raw fresh fruits and vegetables, wheat grass juice (can be replaced with green food supplements), water and meal replacement shakes. During the next 14 days (weeks two and three) the patient is instructed to add soaked raw nuts (almonds and sesame seeds) and sprouted grains to his/her diet, continuing to drink meal replacement shakes, wheat grass juice and water. The program also involves the systematic re-introduction of foods into the diet after the 21 day period to aid in addressing any potential food allergenicities that the practitioner may want to address after the conclusion of the purification protocol. Mental, emotional and spiritual cleansing also occurs during this program. The program additionally requires that the patient practice complimentary methods of purification including colon irrigation, systemic hydrotherapy, lymphatic massage and skin brushing. The supplement and meal replacement recommendations are identical to Program One.

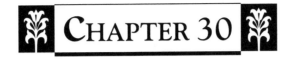

CHAPTER 30

CLINICAL PURIFICATION™ PROTOCOL PROGRAM ONE

INTENSITY : MILD

"The natural force within each one of us is the greatest healer of disease."
—Hippocrates

30

-->X<--

CLINICAL PURIFICATION™ PROTOCOL PROGRAM ONE

INTENSITY : MILD

Overeating and Disease

You can't pick up a magazine, turn on the television, or engage in conversation these days without noticing some reference to the subject of eating, weight, or their relationship to health. A strong and growing body of research suggests that our society as a whole, eats too much, eats too much of the wrong kinds of foods, and fails to get adequate exercise. All of this weight-related scrutiny has led to a plethora of dieting fads, supplements, weight-reduction regimens, and "diet foods."

Unfortunately, the focus for the need to cut back on caloric intake is still greatly influenced by the number on the scale, the size of clothing we wear, or how we look. Nevertheless, of far greater importance is the effect of weight on overall health. When we eat more than our bodies use, we begin to gain weight. Excess weight can lead to problems with our skeletal system, increased risk for developing cardiovascular disease, diabetes, metabolic problems, and some cancers. Eating too much can also accelerate the aging process.

Excuses to keep eating too much

Statistics reveal an increasing trend of obesity in our society – even among our children. While we live in an age of global communication and growing health awareness, most of us continue to weigh too much and move too little. We say we don't have time to exercise. We say we're stressed out, lonely, frustrated, tired, depressed, have too many social commitments that involve food, don't know which diets work, find the multitude of diet literature out there confusing, or any other reason we can find to justify eating too much. However, continuing to make excuses for why we eat too much, rather than taking control of the situation may potentially jeopardize our health and affect our quality of life.

No more excuses for eating too much

One of the easiest, safest, and most cost-effective ways to reduce your caloric intake is to do just that – cut your normal portion sizes in half for 21 days. *For example*: Let's say you have a large glass of orange juice, two eggs, and two pieces of toast for breakfast. You don't have to cut out the eggs – eggs are rich in essential macro and micronutrients. But your body will get plenty of nutrients from one egg, instead of two. Do the same thing with the bread. While this is not the "ideal" purification diet, it is realistic and will help to give your detoxification organs a break from the demands of digestion. To help make the transition easier (i.e., prevent those hunger pangs), try to incorporate 1-2 whole food-based supplement shakes into your daily regime as well. They offer you a nutrient-dense balanced source of ingredients that will help to satiate you as well as support your body's detoxification organs. Additionally follow the recommended clinical purification supplement program to support the whole process.

If you're dining out, either look for something that appeals to you that is listed as a smaller portion, for example, a half of a sandwich instead of a whole one, or, take half of it home. Should you cut out ice cream cones? Get a dish of ice cream and forego the cone. The idea is to cut back, and cut back consistently. Don't eat a huge breakfast and then skip lunch. *Reduce everything that you normally eat by half and try to drink at least 1-2 whole food-based supplement shakes (taken BEFORE your regular meal is best) per day*. Drink at least eight glasses of water every day and remember to exercise regularly. You don't have to run 30 minutes a day to improve your health. Find something you enjoy doing and do it at least three times per week. This can include gentle movements to your favorite music, a 20-minute walk with a good friend to share your thoughts and feelings with, or an easy hike through nature.

Clinical Purification™ Program One - Mild
Your three-week cleansing program in a nutshell

Week One

General

- Cut all your meal portions in half
- Drink a whole food-based supplement shake* before 1-2 of your daily meals
- Exercise at least three times per week, and preferably daily
- Drink at least 8 glasses of water per day
- Consider doing enemas, colon or systemic hydrotherapy, skin brushing or getting lymphatic massages

Supplement Program

Follow a recommended clinical purification supplement program, preferably using products that include the whole food and herbal ingredients outlined in this book, specific for addressing all organs that affect the purification process. Look for cleansing and whole food-based supplemental shake products that have been clinically trialed and consistently demonstrate profound results.**

Weeks Two and Three

General

- Cut all your meal portions in half
- Drink a whole food-based nutritional supplement shake* before 1-2 of your daily meals
- Exercise at least three times per week, but preferably daily
- Drink at least 8 glasses of water per day
- Consider doing enemas, colon or systemic hydrotherapy, skin brushing or getting lymphatic massages

Supplement Program

Follow a supplement regimen that specifically addresses gastrointestinal function. Look for a gastrointestinal/fiber product that includes Psyllium, Apple Pectin, and Fenugreek seeds that is proven clinically effective during a purification program.**

* Recommended Whole Food-Based Nutritional Shake Recipe (Developed by Dr. David Minzel, Ph.D., C.N.C., R.C.)

- 1 scoop of whole food-based shake powder   • 1-2 cups of water
- 1/2 cup of your favorite fresh or frozen organic fruit (examples include berries, banana, peaches, apples, cherries)
- 2 tsp high quality oil (examples include flax seed oil, hemp seed oil or Omega's Essential Oil Balance)

Directions: Blend all ingredients together. Wait a few minutes and then add additional water and/or fruit until you achieve the desired consistency and flavor. You may make a large enough batch to last you 1-2 days, but make sure to keep it refrigerated, and remix it if need be before pouring.

** Minzel, D. et al. 2001. Effect of specific whole food complexes on the enhancement of Phase I and Phase II liver detoxification pathways: An examination of enzyme function in human subjects. *Whole Food Nutr J* 1: 26-37.[1]

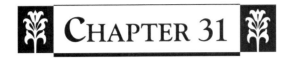

CHAPTER 31

CLINICAL PURIFICATION™ PROTOCOL PROGRAM TWO

INTENSITY : MODERATE

"A wise man should consider that health is the greatest of human blessings…"
– Hippocrates

31

֎֎҉֍֍

CLINICAL PURIFICATION™ PROTOCOL PROGRAM TWO

INTENSITY : MODERATE

Detoxification, digestion, and food sensitivities

While we'd like to believe that almost everything we eat is loaded with nutrients and essential fuel for our bodies, the reality is that processed foods pale in comparison to whole foods when it comes to nutrient density. Packaged foods that we buy in most of our grocery stores contain additives and preservatives. Processing and refining techniques rob precious nutrients, resulting in a finished product that may be devoid of key nutritional factors and the whole food matrix from which they originally came. The food chain has been contaminated with pollutants in the form of pesticides and herbicides, as well as toxic heavy metals, that end up on our produce, and that are stored in the fat cells of our animals.

The second toxic hit our bodies endure happens *inside* the body during the digestive process. Some people experience a strong, acute allergic reaction to foods like milk, peanuts, or shellfish – complete with hives, difficulty, breathing, etc. while others may experience reactions to foods that are less obvious, and can be more chronic in nature. We may be completely unaware that we are sensitive to certain foods, with reactions including headaches, abdominal pain, mood swings, or changes in bowel habits that may be remedied by identifying the cause, eliminating the irritant and improving the functioning of the gastrointestinal tract. For whatever biological reason, we may have less of an intestinal tolerance for certain types of foods, and over time this may tax our detoxification mechanisms and affect our ability to maintain or obtain optimal digestive function.

Cleansing and revitalizing your digestive tract

In order to give your digestive system a break and help your body cleanse itself from the inside out, remove the following food items from your diet for a full 21-day period. Not only will this give your body a rest from digestive irritants, but if you choose to reintroduce these foods into your diet later on, you can do so one at a time. You will soon be able to tell if you are sensitive to a particular food by the way that you feel – your body's natural wellness indicator. While on a purification program it is important for you to supplement your diet with nutrient dense foods and herbs that support all of the organs in your body that take part in the purification process.

What foods you should stop eating

For the next three weeks, refrain from eating any:

- wheat (only exception, organic sprouted wheat berries)
- dairy products
- hydrogenated oils
- refined sugars
- vinegar (except apple cider vinegar)
- caffeine (coffee, non-herbal iced tea, etc.)
- carbonated beverages
- eggs
- chicken or red meat (if you eat any meat, eat only wild game or hormone-free lamb).

If you are still hungry, increase your intake of whole food-based supplement shakes*, fresh fruits, vegetables, and plenty of water – at least eight glasses per day. *Tip*: Squeeze some organic lemon into your water to add flavor and promote re-hydration. To help keep your body consistently focused toward the goal of purification, choose organically grown produce whenever possible.

What foods you can eat

Become a smart shopper. Read labels and make sure you buy only those foods that contain *none* of the ingredients mentioned in the list above. For example, when you're choosing a type of bread, make sure there is no wheat or refined sugar listed in the ingredients. Any other type of grain is acceptable. The easiest way to find these kinds of foods and to get a better variety is by shopping at a natural foods store. Buy:

- only distilled, filtered, or spring water
- fresh fruits and vegetables – organically grown, if possible
- brown, Thai, wild, or basmati rice
- rice-based foods, for example, rice cakes, crackers, bread made with rice flour, pasta, pancake mix, etc.
- non-medicinal herbal or green teas
- bottled fruit and vegetable juices, made from organically grown sources
- unheated cold-pressed flaxseed oil, hemp seed oil or oil blend that is high in essential fatty acids, and olive oil.

Here are some names of smaller companies that are well recognized for high-quality organic foods:

Pasta: Eden, Westbrae, DeBoles, Mendocino Pasta Company

Juices: Santa Cruz, Knudsen, Mountain Sun, Tree of Life

Flour: Shiloh Farms, Arrowhead Mills

Oils: Flora, Spectrum, Barlean's, Omega

Bread: Alvarado, Shiloh Farms, Breads for Life, Garden of Eatin', Food for Life (Ezekiel bread), French Meadow, Nature's Path

Mental/emotional cleansing

Going through a clinical purification program definitely impacts your physical health, but as an added benefit, it also provides you with the opportunity to "clear out" some of the mental and emotional "stuff" that may be slowing you down. As you place less of a strain on your physical body by mindfully eating nutrient dense foods while supporting your body's natural purification process with key whole food based nutrient complexes, you will likely find that your thoughts are clearer and you are better able to handle stress. This transformation welcomes the opportunity to look at, and release any excess baggage that may be keeping you from feeling optimal health. Take a walk with an old friend and share your thoughts, experiences and feelings with him or her. Keep a journal and write down what you are feeling. Talk to a health counselor that you trust. Do whatever you feel comfortable and safe doing that will facilitate your emotional, mental and even spiritual transformation.

Clinical Purification™ Program Two - Moderate
Your three-week cleansing program in a nutshell

Week One

General

- Avoid/include foods as specified above
- Drink a whole food-based supplement shake* before 2-3 of your daily meals
- Exercise and sweat daily   • Drink at least 8 glasses of water per day
- Consider doing enemas, colon or systemic hydrotherapy, skin brushing or getting lymphatic massages
- Mindfully address any mental, emotional or spiritual "issues" that come up

Supplement Program

Follow a recommended clinical purification supplement program, preferably using products that include the whole food and herbal ingredients outlined in this book, that are specific for addressing all organs that affect the purification process. Look for cleansing and meal replacement products that have been clinically trialed and consistently demonstrate profound results.**

Weeks Two and Three

General

- Avoid/include foods as specified above
- Drink a whole food-based supplement shake* before 2-3 of your daily meals
- Exercise daily   • Drink at least 8 glasses of water per day
- Consider doing enemas, colon or systemic hydrotherapy, skin brushing or getting lymphatic massages
- Mindfully address any mental, emotional or spiritual "issues" that come up

Supplement Program

Follow a supplement regimen that specifically addresses gastrointestinal function. Look for a gastrointestinal/fiber product that includes Psyllium, Apple Pectin, and Fenugreek seeds that is proven clinically effective during a purification program.**

---

* Recommended Whole Food-Based Nutritional Shake Recipe (Developed by Dr. David Minzel, Ph.D., C.N.C., R.C.)
- 1 scoop of whole food-based shake powder   • 1-2 cups of water
- 1/2 cup of your favorite fresh or frozen organic fruit (examples include berries, banana, peaches, apples, cherries)
- 2 tsp high quality oil (examples include flax seed oil, hemp seed oil or Omega's Essential Oil Balance)

Directions: Blend all ingredients together. Wait a few minutes and then add additional water and/or fruit until you achieve the desired consistency and flavor. You may make a large enough batch to last you 1-2 days, but make sure to keep it refrigerated, and remix it if need be before pouring.

** Minzel, D. et al. 2001. Effect of specific whole food complexes on the enhancement of Phase I and Phase II liver detoxification pathways: An examination of enzyme function in human subjects. *Whole Food Nutr J* 1: 26-37.[1]

Purification
Protocols
Moderate

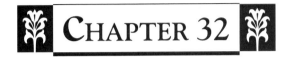

CHAPTER 32

CLINICAL PURIFICATION™ PROTOCOL PROGRAM THREE

INTENSITY : OPTIMAL

*"Hold to that knowledge- and don't think of it as just theory -
that the body can the body does renew itself."*
—Cayce

32

᎞>>҉Κ<᎞

CLINICAL PURIFICATION™ PROTOCOL PROGRAM THREE

INTENSITY : OPTIMAL

The modified fast

O ne of the best ways to rid your body of toxins, rest your digestive system, and promote total body cleansing and rejuvenation is to remove digestive irritants from your diet for a full 21-day period while supplementing your diet with nutrient dense foods and herbs that support the organs in your body that take part in the purification process. While this approach requires a strong commitment and willingness to endure temptation and occasional feelings of hunger and weakness, your reward will be a healthier, more energetic and happier you. This positive change will encourage a healthier lifestyle.

The modified fast removes digestive-system irritants and replaces them with food sources that are cleansing, soothing, and high in chlorophyll content. Wheat grass, for example, is well recognized for its cleansing properties and for its ability to relieve gastric distress. It is also loaded with vital nutrients. Wheat grass contains vitamins A and B12, a protein content as robust as many meats, digestive enzymes, and depending upon the soil it comes from, can hold as many as 90 plus minerals. Wheat grass is highly concentrated and as little as one ounce will produce a beneficial effect. You may experience a mild reaction to wheat grass (diarrhea, headache, or other symptoms), but these symptoms usually occur only a few times during a purification process, and can be a sign that your detoxification mechanisms are kicking in.

What to eat – Week one

For the first seven days of your purification regimen, eat only:

- *raw* fruits and vegetables
- Whole Food-Based Supplement Shakes*

Drink two ounces of wheat grass juice daily. *Caution:* As is often the case, more is not better. Stick with the two-ounce serving size because as mentioned above, wheat grass is very concentrated and taking more will not increase efficacy. *Tip:* If wheat grass juice is not available to you, substitute with a whole food-based green food supplement (place approximately 2.5 grams of powder- usually equates to about 7-8 capsules- in 8 oz of water).

What to eat – Weeks Two and Three

For days 8 through 21 eat only:

- *raw* fruits and vegetables
- *raw* almonds and sesame seeds soaked and rinsed in distilled water- soak for at least six hours or overnight in the refrigerator then rinse with distilled water.
- *sprouted* grains
- Whole Food-Based Supplement Shakes*

Continue drinking two ounces of wheat grass juice each day, or substitute with a whole food-based green food supplement (place approximately 2.5 grams of powder- usually about 7-8 capsules- in 8 oz of water).

Remember: Eat only the foods listed in each seven or fourteen-day period – no substitutions. This diet is specifically formulated to offer the greatest purification benefit in tandem with optimal nutrition.

Shopping tips

Become a smart shopper. The easiest way to find these kinds of foods and to get a better variety is by shopping at a natural foods store. Buy:

- only distilled, filtered, or spring water
- fresh fruits and vegetables – organically grown, if possible

Maintaining good nutrition and hydration during the purification process

Throughout your 21-day detoxifying regimen, make sure you take the recommended dietary supplements to ensure adequate supplies of all essential nutrients. Drink at least eight full glasses of distilled, filtered, or spring water every day. Water is involved in almost every bodily process, is the primary vehicle for distributing nutrients throughout the body, helps maintain normal body temperature, and transports waste material out of the body.

The re-entry phase

Your 21-day detoxifying regimen was designed to cleanse your entire body from internal and external toxins, and give your digestive system a therapeutic rest. Your digestive system will react negatively if instantly bombarded with all kinds of digestive irritants on day 22. It is important to re-introduce solid foods slowly into the daily diet. And, since your system is virtually "clean" from all food allergens at this point, it is an excellent time to assess which foods your body finds mildly irritating.

Remember: Report any adverse reactions to your healthcare practitioner. He or she will be able to tell you whether you're feeling a normal reaction to your detoxification/re-entry regimen or whether you need medical attention.

Suggested re-entry schedule

You may have thought throughout the past 21 days that you just couldn't wait to sink your teeth into a nice greasy cheeseburger, a chocolate éclair, or any type of food you've always considered you couldn't live without. Nevertheless, once your body is accustomed to living without all of these digestive irritants, the cravings for them subside proportionately. As you re-introduce certain foods into your diet over a period of time, you'll be able to tell within a couple of days which foods irritate your digestive system. You'll then be able to either cut down on the offenders or delete them from your diet completely, so you can feel much better all of the time.

- Eat raw fruits and some steamed vegetables the *first day* of your re-entry phase.
- Add white rice to your diet on *day two* of your re-entry phase.
- If desired, add wild game, lamb, and legumes on *day three* of the re-entry phase.

Now you are ready to begin *allergen testing*. It takes approximately three days to monitor your body's reaction to a certain food. If you can tolerate them after three days, you can continue eating them. If you find you just don't feel right, it's time to decide whether or not to include them and to what extent, in your daily diet.

Add *one* potential allergen every three days, beginning on the fourth day of your re-entry phase. Try eating:

- dairy products for three days and see how you feel.
- wheat products for three days and see how you feel.
- sugar products for three days and see how you feel.
- eggs for three days and see how you feel.
- corn products for three days and see how you feel.
- soy products for three days and see how you feel.
- peanuts for three days and see how you feel.

Now you have a clear indication from observing your body's reactions to these specific foods, which foods it can digest easily and which foods irritate your gastrointestinal tract.

Mental/emotional cleansing

Going through a clinical purification program definitely impacts your physical health, but as an added benefit, it also provides you with the opportunity to "clear out" some of the mental and emotional "stuff" that may be slowing you down. As you place less of a strain on your physical body by mindfully eating nutrient dense foods while supporting your body's natural purification process with key whole food-based nutrient complexes, you will likely find that your thoughts are clearer and you are better able to handle stress. This transformation welcomes the opportunity to look at, and release any excess baggage that may be keeping you from feeling optimal health. Take a walk with an old friend and share your thoughts, experiences and feelings with him or her. Keep a journal and write down what you are feeling. Talk to a health counselor that you trust. Do whatever you feel comfortable and safe doing that will facilitate your emotional, mental and even spiritual transformation.

While you've heard them all before, the following recommendations are an investment in your good health and longevity. They are both inexpensive and give you total control of your basic health care, and will help you change your habits for life.

- Find an activity you enjoy and do it for 20 minutes each day.

- Give your mind a rest. Find a hobby, read, listen to music, or do whatever reduces stress for you and helps you reverse negative energy.

- Keep drinking at least eight full glasses of clean water every day.

- Take natural, whole-food based, dietary supplements.

- Eat healthy and balanced meals regularly.

- Get enough sleep. Most people require eight hours per night of sleep in order to feel physically refreshed and mentally sharp each day.

Clinical Purification™ Program Three - Optimal
Your three-week cleansing program in a nutshell

Week One
General

- Eat fresh, raw, organic (if possible) fruits and vegetables, particularly green leafy vegetables (kale, spinach, dandelion, etc.)
- Avoid all other foods   • Drink a whole food-based supplement shake* whenever you are hungry
- Drink two ounces of wheat grass juice each day, or substitute with a whole food-based green food supplement (place approximately 2.5 grams of powder- usually about 7-8 capsules- in 8 oz of water).
- Exercise and sweat daily   • Drink at least 8 glasses of water per day
- Mindfully address any mental, emotional or spiritual "issues" that come up
- Consider doing enemas, colon or systemic hydrotherapy, skin brushing or getting lymphatic massages

Supplement Program

Follow a recommended clinical purification supplement program, preferably using products that include the whole food and herbal ingredients outlined in this book, that are specific for addressing all organs that affect the purification process. Look for cleansing and meal replacement products that have been clinically trialed and consistently demonstrate profound results.**

Weeks Two and Three
General

- eat only: • raw fruits and vegetables   • soaked raw almonds and sesame seeds   • sprouted grains
- Continue drinking two ounces of wheat grass juice each day, or substitute a whole food-based green food supplement (place approximately 2.5 grams of powder- usually about 7-8 capsules- in 8 oz of water).
- Drink a whole food-based supplement shake* before 2-3 of your daily meals
- Exercise daily   • Drink at least 8 glasses of water per day
- Mindfully address any mental, emotional or spiritual "issues" that come up
- Consider doing enemas, colonics, skin brushing, getting a massage or practicing hydrotherapy as needed

Supplement Program

Follow a supplement regimen that specifically addresses gastrointestinal function. Look for a gastrointestinal/fiber product that includes Psyllium, Apple Pectin, and Fenugreek seeds that is proven clinically effective during a purification program.**

---

* Recommended Whole Food-Based Nutritional Shake Recipe (Developed by Dr. David Minzel, Ph.D., C.N.C., R.C.)
- 1 scoop of whole food-based shake powder   • 1-2 cups of water
- 1/2 cup of your favorite fresh or frozen organic fruit (examples include berries, banana, peaches, apples, cherries)
- 2 tsp high quality oil (examples include flax seed oil, hemp seed oil or Omega's Essential Oil Balance)

Directions: Blend all ingredients together. Wait a few minutes and then add additional water and/or fruit until you achieve the desired consistency and flavor. You may make a large enough batch to last you 1-2 days, but make sure to keep it refrigerated, and remix it if need be before pouring.

** Minzel, D. et al. 2001. Effect of specific whole food complexes on the enhancement of Phase I and Phase II liver detoxification pathways: An examination of enzyme function in human subjects. *Whole Food Nutr J* 1: 26-37.[1]

PART 4
CLINICAL REFERENCES

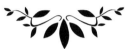

(CHAPTERS 30-32)

1. Anderson, D.A., et al. Estimation of food intake: effects of the unit of estimation. *Eating and Weight Disorders*. 1999. Mar;4(1):6-9.
2. Asero, R., et al. Lipid transfer protein: A pan-allergen in plant-derived foods that is highly resistant to pepsin digestion. *International Archives of Allergy and Immunology*. 2000. May;122(1):20-32.
3. Astrup, A., et al. The role of dietary fat in body fatness: evidence from a preliminary meta-analysis of ad libitum low-fat dietary intervention studies. *British Journal of Nutrition*. 2000. Mar;83 Suppl 1:S25-32.
4. Balch, James F., M.D. and Balch, Phyllis A., C.N.C. *Prescription for Nutritional Healing*, 2nd ed. 1993. Avery Publishing Group, Garden City Park, NY. pps.30-3,61.
5. Eigenmann, P.A. and Calza, A.M. Diagnosis of IgE-mediated food allergy among Swiss children with atopic dermatitis. *Pediatric Allergy and Immunology*. 2000. May;11(2):95-100.
6. Folsom, A.R., et al. Associations of General and Abdominal Obesity With Multiple Health Outcomes in Older Women: The Iowa Women's Health Study. *Archives of Internal Medicine*. 2000. Jul 24;160(14):2117-28.
7. Greenwald, P. and McDonald, S.S. Cancer Prevention: The Roles of Diet and Chemoprevention. *Cancer Control*. 1997. Mar;4(2):118-27.
8. Impellizeri, J.A., et al. Effect of weight reduction on clinical signs of lameness in dogs with hip osteoarthritis. *Journal of the American Veterinary Association*. 2000. Apr 1;216(7):1089-91.
9. Lichtenstein, A.H., et.al. Effects of different forms of dietary hydrogenated fats on serum lipoprotein cholesterol levels. *New England Journal of Medicine*. 1999. Jun 24;340(25):1933-40.
10. Lichtenstein, A.H. Dietary trans fatty acids. *Journal of Cardiopulmonary Rehabilitation*. 2000. May-Jun;20(3):143-6.
11. Mangweth, B., et al. Knowledge of calories and its effect on eating behavior in overweight, normal weight, and underweight individuals. *Eating and Weight Disorders*. 1999. Dec;4(4):165-8.
12. McKelvey, W., et al. A second look at the relation between colorectal adenomas and consumption of foods containing partially hydrogenated oils. *Epidemiology*. 2000. Jul;11(4):469-73.
13. Minzel, D. et al. 2001. Effect of specific whole food complexes on the enhancement of Phase I and Phase II liver detoxification pathways: An examination of enzyme function in human subjects. 1(1): 26-37.
14. Moneret-Vautrin, D.A., et al. [The multifood allergy syndrome]. *Allergy and Immunology* (Paris). 2000. Jan;32(1):12-5.
15. Pelto, L., et al. Milk hypersensitivity in young adults. *European Journal of Clinical Nutrition*. 1999. Aug;53(8):620-4.
16. Pitchford, Paul. *Healing With Whole Foods*. Revised ed. 1993. North Atlantic Books, Berekely, CA. pps.75-9. 199-206, 232-3.
17. Serdula, M.K., et al. Prevalence of attempting weight loss and strategies for controlling weight. *JAMA*. 1999. Oct 13;282(14):1353-8.
18. Stone, N.J., and Kushner, R. Effects of dietary modification and treatment of obesity. Emphasis on improving vascular outcomes. *Med Clin North Am*. 2000. Jan;84(1):95-122.
19. Yance, Donald R., Jr., C.N., M.H., A.H/G., with Valentine, Arlene. *Herbal Medicine, Healing & Cancer*. 1999. Keats Publishing, Division of NTC/Contemporary Publishing Group, Inc. Lincolnwood, IL. p.73, 354-5.

APPENDIX A

TOXICITY QUESTIONNAIRE

PATIENT HANDOUT

Toxicity Questionnaire

The Toxicity Questionnaire is designed to aid the practitioner in assessing a
patient or client's potential need for a Clinical Purification™ program

Section I: Symptoms

Rate each of the following symptoms based upon your health profile for the past 90 days.

Circle the corresponding number.	
0	Rarely or Never Experience the Symptom
1	Occasionally Experience the Symptom, Effect **is not** Severe
2	Occasionally Experience the Symptom, Effect **is** Severe
3	Frequently Experience the Symptom, Effect **is not** Severe
4	Frequently Experience the Symptom, Effect **is** Severe

1. DIGESTIVE

a. Nausea and/or vomiting	0	1	2	3	4
b. Diarrhea	0	1	2	3	4
c. Constipation	0	1	2	3	4
d. Bloated feeling	0	1	2	3	4
e. Belching and/or passing gas	0	1	2	3	4
f. Heartburn	0	1	2	3	4
Total					

2. EARS

a. Itchy ears	0	1	2	3	4
b. Earaches, ear infections	0	1	2	3	4
c. Drainage from ear	0	1	2	3	4
d. Ringing in ears, hearing loss	0	1	2	3	4
Total					

3. EMOTIONS

a. Mood swings	0	1	2	3	4
b. Anxiety, fear, nervousness	0	1	2	3	4
c. Anger, irritability	0	1	2	3	4
d. Depression	0	1	2	3	4
e. Sense of despair	0	1	2	3	4
f. Apathy/ lethargy	0	1	2	3	4
Total					

4. ENERGY/ACTIVITY

a. Fatigue / sluggishness	0	1	2	3	4
b. Hyperactivity	0	1	2	3	4
c. Restlessness	0	1	2	3	4
d. Insomnia	0	1	2	3	4
e. Startled awake at night	0	1	2	3	4
Total					

5. EYES

a. Watery, itchy eyes	0	1	2	3	4
b. Swollen, reddened or sticky eyelids	0	1	2	3	4
c. Dark circles under eyes	0	1	2	3	4
d. Blurred/tunnel vision	0	1	2	3	4
Total					

6. HEAD

a. Headaches	0	1	2	3	4
b. Faintness	0	1	2	3	4
c. Dizziness	0	1	2	3	4
d. Pressure	0	1	2	3	4
Total					

7. LUNGS

a. Chest congestion	0	1	2	3	4
b. Asthma, Bronchitis	0	1	2	3	4
c. Shortness of breath	0	1	2	3	4
d. Difficulty breathing	0	1	2	3	4
Total					

8. MIND

a. Poor memory	0	1	2	3	4
b. Confusion	0	1	2	3	4
c. Poor concentration	0	1	2	3	4
d. Poor coordination	0	1	2	3	4
e. Difficulty making decisions	0	1	2	3	4
f. Stuttering, stammering	0	1	2	3	4
g. Slurred speech	0	1	2	3	4
h. Learning disabilities	0	1	2	3	4
Total					

9. MOUTH / THROAT

a. Chronic coughing	0	1	2	3	4
b. Gagging, frequent need to clear throat	0	1	2	3	4
c. Swollen or discolored tongue, gums, lips	0	1	2	3	4
d. Canker sores	0	1	2	3	4
Total					

10. NOSE

a. Stuffy nose	0	1	2	3	4
b. Sinus problems	0	1	2	3	4
c. Hay fever	0	1	2	3	4
d. Sneezing attacks	0	1	2	3	4
e. Excessive mucous	0	1	2	3	4
Total					

11. SKIN

a. Acne	0	1	2	3	4
b. Hives, rashes, dry skin	0	1	2	3	4
c. Hair loss	0	1	2	3	4
d. Flushing	0	1	2	3	4
e. Excessive sweating	0	1	2	3	4
Total					

12. HEART

a. Skipped heartbeats	0	1	2	3	4
b. Rapid heartbeats	0	1	2	3	4
c. Chest pain	0	1	2	3	4
Total					

13. JOINTS / MUSCLES

a. Pain or aches in joints	0	1	2	3	4
b. Rheumatoid arthritis	0	1	2	3	4
c. Osteoarthritis	0	1	2	3	4
d. Stiffness, limited movement	0	1	2	3	4
e. Pain, aches in muscles	0	1	2	3	4
f. Recurrent back aches	0	1	2	3	4
g. Feeling of weakness or tiredness	0	1	2	3	4
Total					

14. WEIGHT

a. Binge eating/drinking	0	1	2	3	4
b. Craving certain foods	0	1	2	3	4
c. Excessive weight	0	1	2	3	4
d. Compulsive eating	0	1	2	3	4
e. Water retention	0	1	2	3	4
f. Underweight	0	1	2	3	4
Total					

15. OTHER

a. Frequent illness	0	1	2	3	4
b. Frequent or urgent urination	0	1	2	3	4
c. Leaky bladder	0	1	2	3	4
d. Genital itch, discharge	0	1	2	3	4
Total					

Section I Total _____

Handout
Toxicity
Questionnaire

Section II: Risk of Exposure

Rate each of the following situations based upon your environmental profile for the past 120 days.

16.	Circle the corresponding number for questions 16a-f below.

0 Never	**1** Rarely	**2** Monthly	**3** Weekly	**4** Daily

a. How often are strong chemicals used in your home ? (disinfectants, bleaches, oven and drain cleaners, furniture polish, floor wax, window cleaners, etc.)	0 1 2 3 4
b. How often are pesticides used in your home?	0 1 2 3 4
c. How often do you have your home treated for insects?	0 1 2 3 4
d. How often are you exposed to dust, overstuffed furniture, tobacco smoke, mothballs, incense or varnish in your home or office?	0 1 2 3 4
e. How often are you exposed to nail polish, perfume, hair spray and other cosmetics?	0 1 2 3 4
f. How often are you exposed to diesel fumes, exhaust fumes, or gasoline fumes?	0 1 2 3 4

Total _____

17.	Circle the corresponding number for questions 17a-b below.

0 No	**1** Mild Change	**2** Moderate Change	**3** Drastic Change

a. Have you noticed any negative change in your health since you moved into your home or apartment?	0 1 2 3
b. Have you noticed any negative change in your health since you started your new job?	0 1 2 3

Total _____

18.	Answer yes or no and circle the corresponding number for questions 18a-d below.

	No	Yes
a. Do you have a water purification system in your home?	2	0
b. Do you have any indoor pets?	0	2
c. Do you have an air purification system in your home?	2	0
d. Are you a dentist, painter, farm worker or construction worker?	0	2

Total _____

GRAND TOTAL (Section I + Section II) _____

Add up the numbers to arrive at a total for each section, and then add the totals for each section to arrive at the grand total. If any individual section total is 6 or more, or the grand total is 40 or more, you may benefit from a Clinical Purification™ program.

APPENDIX B

Sixteen Vital Principles to Live by for Optimal Health

PATIENT HANDOUT

16 Vital Principles to Live by for Optimal Health

1. Avoid eating if you feel stressed or anxious.

2. Listen to your body - don't eat if you're not hungry, and conversely, don't put up with hunger pains. Stop eating once you begin to feel full and no longer have an appetite.

3. Drink 8 to 12 glasses of filtered water daily. Avoid large amounts of fluid with meals.

4. Avoid eating large amounts of sugar - especially refined sugars.

5. Avoid caffeine.

6. Avoid foods you may be allergic to.

7. Chew your food slowly.

8. Limit your intake, and if possible avoid packaged and processed foods containing artificial chemicals such as preservatives, colorings, flavorings and synthetic sweeteners.

9. Try to eat organically grown fresh produce, free of pesticides and herbicides.

10. Try to eat organically-reared animal products, stay clear of reheated meats and always buy free-range eggs.

11. Obtain your protein from diverse sources (including legumes) not just from animal products such as meat, eggs and fish - you can obtain first-class protein by combining in one meal any three of the four following foods - grains (wheat, buckwheat, rice, barley, rye, oats, millet etc.), nuts, seeds and legumes.

12. Choose your breads wisely - it is important to eat only good quality breads, which provide fiber, minerals and the B and E vitamin complexes. Most bread you find today is made by mass production methods using ingredients like hydrogenated vegetable oils, monoacetyltartaric acid, disodium dihydrogen diphosphate, and other artificial chemicals.

13. Avoid constipation - eat plenty of raw fruits and vegetables and drink plenty of water during the day. Supplement with a whole food based gastrointestinal purification product.

14. Avoid excessive saturated or hydrogenated fats and incorporate essential fatty acid oil blends into your diet as a replacement. Recommended oils include cold pressed organic hemp seed oil, flax seed oil, and Essential Oil Balance by Omega.

15. Help someone out, no matter how small or grand the task, each day.

16. Smile…Laugh

APPENDIX C

Directions for Administering an Enema

PATIENT HANDOUT

Directions for Administering an Enema

Enema bags or colema boards are useful tools for cleansing your colon at home. The enema bag is cheaper than a colema board, holds much less water (thus less water gets into the colon), and is not done over the toilet, whereas a colema board is done over the toilet.

Hang the enema bag at least 18 inches above your body. Before you fill the bag, make sure the tubing clamp is shut tight so that the content of the bag does not leak out. Fill the bag with warm (comfortable to touch), purified, distilled or reverse osmosis water. Lubricate the rectal tip with a non-petroleum lubricant like vitamin E. Lie on your back on a towel on the floor, or even in a tepid water bath and insert the rectal tip. Open the tubing clamp. Let as much liquid into your colon as you feel comfortable with and then re-clamp the tubing. At this point, either massage your colon from left to right, descending colon to ascending colon, in small circular motions or lift your buttocks off the ground with your legs to further move the liquid into your colon. Try to retain the enema for about 15 minutes or longer. Evacuate whenever you need to.

Make sure you haven't ingested anything for 2 hours prior to starting the enema. After you complete your enema, wait at least 45 minutes before ingesting anything.

Colema Boards are more expensive, hold 4-5 gallons of water and are done over the toilet. You fill the bucket with room temperature, reverse osmosis water. It must sit one to two feet above your body. You will have to get suction in the hose before it will flow down. To do this, fill the plastic hose up with water and let some of it out. This will create suction. Clamp the tube and put one end in the bucket.

One end of the colema board lies over the toilet bowl and the other end lies on a chair. Place one or two towels on the board for comfort. Lubricate the plastic tubing which goes into the rectum. Lie down and insert the tube into the rectum. Allow the water to follow into your colon. At first, do not try to hold too much water. If you feel any pressure, then simply "let go" and the water will come pouring out into the toilet. The more you get used to taking home colonics, the more you will know exactly how much you can hold.

Some people feel much more at ease having a trained professional assisting them to clean their colon. When that is the case, consider going to a colon hydrotherapist for a professional colonic treatment.

Enema Recipe

Olive Oil/Aloe Vera: In an enema bag, pour one cup of organic olive oil and one cup of organic aloe vera juice. Open four whole food-based fiber capsules and mix with liquid. Slowly pour into colon with enema bag. Hold as long as you are able. This will soothe the intestinal lining during inflammation as well as clean the colon.

Handout
Administering
an Enema

APPENDIX D

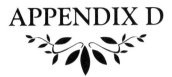

Modified Constitutional Hydrotherapy Guidelines

PATIENT HANDOUT

Modified Constitutional Hydrotherapy Guidelines

This modified Constitutional Hydrotherapy technique involves a series of hot and cold compress applications to the chest, abdomen and back.

Materials:

Two 100% wool blankets

One pillow

Massage or treatment table (preferable but not required)

Four bath-sized towels

Sink or bucket filled with ice cubes and cold water

Sink or bucket filled with hot water

Guidelines for Treatment:

1. Place one wool blanket length wise along the treatment table with one pillow at head of table.

2. Instruct patient to undress from the waist up, lie face up on the table and cover him/herself with the other blanket.

3. Soak two towels in hot water and wring enough so that they do not drip. Test the towels on the wrist to assure that they do not burn the patient.

4. Expose the patient's chest and abdomen and place the hot towels, one directly upon the other, slowly, over the chest and abdomen. Cover the patient immediately with the blanket and wait 5 minutes.

5. During that time, prepare one cold towel by soaking it in an ice water bath and gently ring out so that it does not drip, and prepare one hot towel as done previously.

6. After 5 minutes, open the patient's blanket and place the new hot towel upon the two towels that are already there. Quickly flip all three towels over so that the new hot towel is now on the patient's skin. Remove the other two towels.

7. Immediately place the cold towel over the new hot towel and again flip both towels so that the cold towel is now touching the patient.

8. Quickly remove the hot towel and cover the patient completely with the blanket.

9. Wait ten minutes and then check to see if the patient has warmed the previously cold towel. If not, wait another 3 minutes and re-check. If the towel is warm, remove it and have the patient turn over, face down. If the towel fails to warm, repeat until the patient is able to warm the towel.

10. Repeat the entire process on the backside.

APPENDIX E

Dry Skin Brushing

PATIENT HANDOUT

Dry Skin Brushing

As the largest eliminative organ, the skin plays a vital role in ridding the body of toxins. As part of the Clinical Purification™ process, healthcare practitioners can recommend dry skin brushing to their patients to open up the pores of the skin and support lymphatic cleansing. When the pores are not clogged with dead cells and the lymphatic system is cleansed, the body is able to carry out the function of eliminating toxins and waste material.

How to Skin Brush

It is important to practice dry skin brushing every day during the Clinical Purification™ process. The best time to dry skin brush is upon rising, prior to showering, when the skin is completely dry. The brush, which must be completely dry, is a natural vegetable-bristle brush with a long handle to aid in brushing hard- to- reach areas of the body. Begin by gently brushing with one-stroke movements. If the skin reddens, the patient is brushing too hard. The basic principle is to brush from the outermost points of one's body (hands and feet) towards the center. Start by brushing from the feet to the abdomen, then from the hands up to the arms towards the heart. Brush across the upper back and down the front and back of the torso. One should aim to cover the entire surface of the skin. The process takes between three and five minutes to complete.

Overview

Dry skin brushing is a useful adjunctive therapy that helps to release toxins from the body.

Additionally, the process of dry skin brushing:

- Boosts immune function

- Stimulates the lymphatic system

- Stimulates the circulatory system.

Handout
Dry Skin
Brushing

APPENDIX F

Yoga and Breathing

PATIENT HANDOUT

YOGA AND BREATHING

The word "yoga" is derived from the verbal root, yuj, meaning to yoke or harness. Yoga is the process of unifying one's mind body and soul in order to express the energy of one's true nature. In the author's professional opinion, based on personal experience with practicing and teaching yoga, hatha yoga (a type of yoga referred to as "physical" yoga) is the ideal exercise practice while going through a clinical purification program. *Just as one uses alchemic principles to create a purification formula from herbs and foods to address the functioning of specific organs in the body, hatha yoga involves the alchemic reprogramming of mind and body that serves to release toxins and purify the soul.*

The word "hatha" is derived from the Sanskrit root, ha (sun) and tha (moon), and is the equalization and stabilization of the sun-moon (yin-yang) life-force. The purpose of Hatha yoga is to free the body and mind from dysfunctional blockages. With respect to the Clinical Purification™ Process, this equates to the elimination of exogenous and endogenous toxins. Hatha yoga involves a methodical and integrative approach to stretching and contracting different muscle groups to strengthen and lengthen opposing muscles. Hatha also re-aligns the skeleton and applies weight to vital bones to maintain and increase bone density. At the same time and perhaps less obviously, Hatha yoga also gently massages all internal organs.

Following is a series of basic yoga postures that one can begin practicing at home. It is important to be in a warm room, with comfortable clothes and preferably barefoot. When practicing these postures, one must be mindful of his/her body, backing off when one feels pain and slowly extending beyond the point of resistance only when one feels ready to do so. Those who practice yoga regularly often notice a gradual increase in strength, flexibility and balance. *The most critical factor when practicing yoga is to be mindful of one's breath.*

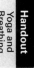

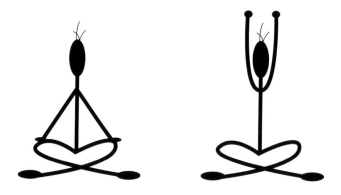

Sit / Easy Position - Sukhasana

A starting position that helps focus awareness on breathing and the body; helps strengthen lower back and open the groin and hips.

Sit cross-legged with hands on knees. Focus on your breath. Keep your spine straight and push the sit bones down into the floor. Allow the knees to gently lower. If the knees rise above your hips, sit on a cushion or block. This will help support your back and hips. Take 5-10 slow, deep breaths. On the next inhale, raise your arms over your head. Exhale and bring your arms down slowly. Repeat 5-7 times.

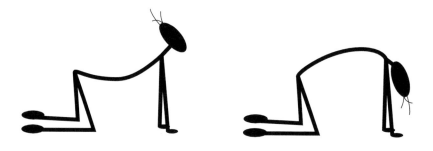

Dog and Cat

Increases flexibility of the spine.

Begin on your hands and knees. Keep your hands just in front of your shoulders, your legs about hip width apart. As you inhale, tilt the tailbone and pelvis up, and let the spine curve downward, dropping the stomach low, and lift your head up. Stretch gently. As you exhale, move into cat by reversing the spinal bend, tilting the pelvis down, drawing the spine up and pulling the chest and stomach in. Repeat several times, flowing smoothly from dog into cat, and cat back into dog.

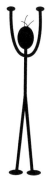

Mountain - Tadasana

Improves posture, balance and self-awareness.

Stand with feet together, hands at your sides, eyes looking forward. Raise your toes, fan them open, then place them back down on the floor. Feel your heel, outside of your foot, toes and ball of your foot all in contact with the floor. Tilt your pubic bone slightly forward. Raise your chest up and out, but within reason - this isn't the army and you're not standing at attention. Raise your head up and lengthen the neck by lifting the base of your skull toward the ceiling. Stretch the pinky on each hand downward, then balance that movement by stretching your index fingers. Push into the floor with your feet and raise your legs, first the calves and then the thighs.

Breathe. Hold the posture, but try not to tense up. Breathe. As you inhale, imagine the breath coming up through the floor, rising through your legs and torso and up into your head. Reverse the process on the exhale and watch your breath as it passes down from your head, through your chest and stomach, legs and feet.

Hold for 5 to 10 breaths, relax and repeat.

On your next inhale, raise your arms over head (Urdhava Hastasana) and hold for several breaths. Lower your arms on an exhale.

As a warm up, try synchronizing the raising and lowering of your arms with your breath - raise, inhale; lower, exhale. Repeat 5 times.

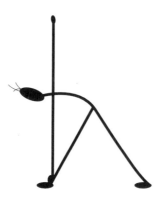

Forward Bend or Extension - Uttanasana II

Stretches the legs and spine, rests the heart and neck, relaxes mind and body

Begin standing straight in Mountain pose or Tadasana. Inhale and raise the arms overhead. Exhale, bend at the hips, bring the arms forward and down until you touch the floor. It's okay to bend your knees, especially if you're feeling stiff. Either grasp your ankles or just leave your hands on the floor and breathe several times. Repeat 3-5 times. On your last bend, hold the position for 5 or 10 breaths. To come out of the pose, curl upward as if pulling yourself up one vertebrae at a time, stacking one on top of another, and leaving the head hanging down until last.

Trikonasana - the Triangle

Stretches the spine, opens the torso, improves balance and concentration.

Start with your legs spread 3-4 feet apart, feet parallel. Turn your left foot 90 degrees to the left and your right foot about 45 degrees inward. Inhale and raise both arms so they're parallel with the floor. Exhale, turn your head to the left and look down your left arm toward your outstretched fingers. Check that your left knee is aligned with your left ankle. Take a deep breath and stretch outward to the left, tilting the left hip down and the right hip up. When you've stretched as far as you can, pivot your arms, letting your left hand reach down and come to rest against the inside of your calf, while your right arms points straight up. Turn and look up at your right hand. Breathe deeply for several breaths. Inhale, and straighten up. Exhale, lower your arms. Put your hands on your hips and pivot on your heels, bringing your feet to face front. Repeat the posture on the other side.

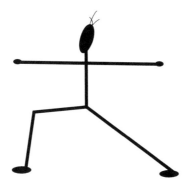

Warrior I I - Virabhadrasana II

Strengthens legs and arms; improves balance and concentration; builds confidence.

Begin in mountain pose with feet together and hands at side. Place your feet 4-5 feet apart. Turn your right foot about 45 degrees to the left. Turn your left foot 90 degrees to the left so that it is pointing straight out to the side. Slowly bend the left knee until the thigh is parallel with the floor, but keep the knee either behind or directly over your ankle. Raise your arms overhead. Then slowly lower them until your left arm is pointing straight ahead and your right arm is pointing back. Concentrate on a spot in front of you and breathe. Take 4 or 5 deep breaths, lower your arms, bring your legs together. Reverse the position.

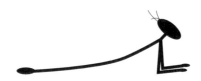

The Cobra - Bhujangasana

Stretches the spine, strengthens the back and arms, opens the chest and heart.

Lay down on your stomach. Keep your legs together, arms at your side, close to your body, with your hands by your chest.

Step 1: Inhaling, slowly raise your head and chest as high as it will go. Keep your buttocks muscles tight to protect your lower back. Keep your head up and chest. Breathe several times and then come down. Repeat as necessary.

Step 2: Follow the steps above. When you've gone as high as you can, gently raise your hands off of the floor stretching the spine even more. Only go as far as you are comfortable. Your pelvis should always remain on the floor. Breathe several times and come down.

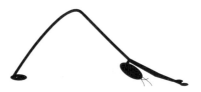

Downward Facing Dog - Adho Mukha Svanasana

Builds strength, flexibility and awareness; stretches the spine and hamstrings; rests the heart.

Start on your hands and knees. Keep your legs about hip width apart and your arms shoulder width apart. Your middle fingers should be parallel, pointing straight ahead. Roll your elbows so that the eye or inner elbow is facing forward. Inhale and curl your toes under, as if getting ready to stand on your toes. Exhale and straighten your legs; push upward with your arms. The goal is to lengthen the spine while keeping your legs straight and your feet flat on the ground. However, in the beginning it's okay to bend the knees a bit and to keep your heels raised. The important thing is to work on lengthening the spine. Don't let your shoulders creep up by your ears - keep them down. Weight should be evenly distributed between your hands and feet. Hold the position for a few breaths. Come down on and exhale. Repeat several times, synchronizing with your breath: up on the exhale and down on the inhale.

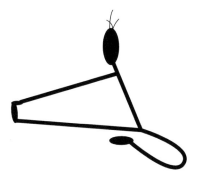

Head to Knee - Janu Shirshasana

Stretches and opens back and hamstrings, improves flexibility

Sit on the floor with legs extended in front of you. Bend one leg, bringing the heel of the foot as close to the groin as possible. You may want to place a pillow under the bent knee for comfort. Make sure your sitz bones are firmly grounded on the floor and that your spine is straight. Turn your body slightly so you face out over the extended leg. Inhale and raise your arms over head. Exhale and begin to move forward slowly. Try to keep the back as straight as possible. Instead of bending at the hips, focus on lifting the tailbone and rolling forward on your sitz bones. Inhale and lengthen and straighten the spine. Exhale and roll forward, however slightly. To get a bit more forward movement, engage your quadriceps (thigh muscles) as you move forward. This releases the hamstrings, giving you a bit more flexibility. When you've moved as far forward as you can, lower the arms and grasp your foot, or leg. Hold the position for a moment and breathe. Then on the next exhale gently pull yourself forward. Go slowly and remember to keep the back straight. When done, straighten up and do the other side.

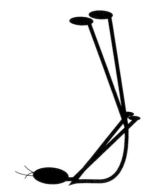

Half Shoulderstand - Ardha Sarvangasana

Promotes proper thyroid function, strengthens abdomen, stretches upper back, improves blood circulation, induces relaxation

You probably remember doing this as a kid. Lie on your back and lift your legs up into air. Place your hands on your lower back for support, resting your elbows and lower arms on the ground. Make sure your weight is on your shoulders and mid to upper back -- not your neck. Breathe deeply and hold for at the posture for at least 5-10 breaths, increasing the hold over time. To come down, slowly lower your legs, keeping them very straight - a little workout for your abdominal muscles.

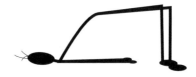

The Bridge - Sethu Bandhasa

Increases flexibility and suppleness; strengthens the lower back and abdominal muscles; opens the chest.

Lay on your back with your knees up and hands at your side Your feet should be near your buttocks about six inches apart. To begin, gently raise and lower your tail. Then, slowly, raise the tailbone and continue lifting the spine, trying to move one vertebra at a time until your entire back is arched upward. Push firmly with your feet. Keep your knees straight and close together. Breathe deeply into your chest. Clasp your hands under your back and push against the floor.

Take five slow, deep breaths.

Come down slowly and repeat.

The Corpse - Savasana

Relaxes and refreshes the body and mind, relieves stress and anxiety, quiets the mind

Possibly the most important posture, the Corpse, is as deceptively simple as Tadasana, the Mountain pose. Usually performed at the end of a session, the goal is conscious relaxation. Many people find the "conscious" part the most difficult because it is very easy to drift off to sleep while doing Savasana. Begin by lying on your back, feet slightly apart, arms at your sides with palms facing up. Close your eyes and take several slow, deep breaths. Allow your body to sink into the ground. Try focusing on a specific part of the body and willing it to relax. For example, start with your feet, imagine the muscles and skin relaxing, letting go and slowly melting into the floor. From your feet, move on to your calves, thighs and so on up to your face and head. Then simply breathe and relax. Stay in the pose for at least 5-10 minutes.

APPENDIX G

RECOMMENDED SOURCES AND ORGANIZATIONS

Professional Organizations and Schools

AAEM
American Academy of Environmental Medicine
7701 East Kellogg, Suite 625
Wichita, Kansas 67207
Tel (316) 684-5500
Fax (316) 684-5709
http://www.aaem.com

AANP
The American Association of Naturopathic Physicians
8201 Greensboro Drive, Suite 300
McLean, VA 22102
Tel (703) 610-9037
Fax (703) 610-9005
http://www.naturopathic.org

Bastyr University
14500 Juanita Drive, NE
Kenmore, WA 98011
Tel (425) 823-1300
Clinic (206) 632-0354
http://www.bastyr.edu

National College of Naturopathic Medicine
049 SW Porter
Portland, OR 97201
Tel (503) 499-4343
Clinic (503) 255-7355
http://www.ncnm.edu

Southwest College of Naturopathic Medicine
and Health Sciences
2140 East Broadway
Tempe, AZ 85282
Tel (480) 858-9100
http://www.scnm.edu

Canadian College of Naturopathic Medicine
1255 Sheppard Avenue, E
North York, ON M2K 1E2
Tel (416) 498-1255
http://www.ccnm.edu

University of Bridgeport
College of Natural Medicine
60 Lafayette Street
Bridgeport, CT 06601
Tel (203) 576-4109
http://www.bridgeport.edu/naturopathy

IFNH
International Foundation for Nutrition and Health
3963 Mission Boulevard
San Diego, CA 92109
Tel (858) 488-8932
http://www.ifnh.org

IACT
International Association for Colon Hydrotherapy
PO Box 461285
San Antonio, TX 78246-1285
Tel (210) 366-2888
Fax (210) 366-2999
iact@healthy.net

Yoga College of India
1862 S. LaCienega Blvd.
Los Angeles, CA 90035
Tel (310) 854-5800
Fax (310) 854-6200
http://www.bikramyoga.com

ACA
American Chiropractic Association
1701 Clarendon Blvd
Arlington, VA 22209
Tel (800) 986-4636
Fax (703) 243-2593
http://www.amerchiro.org

Manual Lymphatic Drainage
Dr. Vodder School
PO Box 5701
Victoria, British Columbia, V8R6S8
Tel (250) 598-9862
Fax (250) 598-9841
http://www.vodderschool.com

Detoxification Institutes

Ann Wigmore Institute
Box 429 Rincon
Puerto Rico 00677 USA
Tel (787) 868-6307
Fax (787) 868-2430

Optimum Health Institute of San Diego
6970 Central Ave.
Lemon Grove, CA 91945-3346
Tel (619) 464-3346
http://www.optimumhealth.org

Optimum Health Institute of Austin
Rt. 1, Box 339-J Cedar Lane
Cedar Creek, TX 78612
Tel (512) 303-4817
Fax (512) 332-0106
http://www.optimumhealth.org

Hippocrates Health Institute
1443 Palmdale Court
West Palm Beach, FL 33411
561-471-8876, 800-842-2125
Fax: 561-471-9464
http://www.hippocratesinst.com

Tree of Life Rejuvenation Center
PO Box 1080, Patagonia, AZ 85624
Tel (520) 394-2520
Fax (520) 394-2099
http://www.treeoflife.nu

Creative Health Institute
918 Union City Road
Union City, MI 49094
Tel (517) 278-6260
e-mail: creative@coldwater.com

Ann Wigmore Foundation
P.O. Box 399
San Fidel, NM 87049
Tel (505) 552-0595
Fax (505) 552-0595
http://www.wigmore.org

Organic Foods

NatuRaw.com
PO Box 18
Fulton, CA 95439-0018
Tel (707) 527-7959
Fax (707) 527-7956
Nationwide delivery of organic foods

Wheatgrass Direct
P.O. Box 249
Ottsville, PA 18942
juiceit@wheatgrassdirect.com
Tel (877) 558-4233 or (610) 346-6687
Fax (610) 346-9478
*Home delivery of fresh, certified organic wheatgrass
and over 25 varieties of sprouts.*

Deer Garden/ Rejuvenative Foods
PO Box 8464
Santa Cruz CA 95060
Tel (831) 457-2418
Fax (831) 457-0158
http://www.rejuvenative.com
*Producers of Organic Raw Cultured Vegetables &
Raw Low Temperature Ground Nut & Seed Butters*

Dave's Organic Produce
35151 Marks Road
Barstow, CA 92311
Tel (760) 256-5339
Fax (760) 252-1241
http://www.davesorganics.com
Organic, Biodynamically Produced Fruits and Vegetables

Diamond Organics
PO Box 2159, Freedom, CA 95019
Tel (888) ORGANIC
Fax (888) 888-6777
http://www.diamondorganics.com
*Fresh, organically grown fruits, vegetables & flowers
shipped direct to your home, year round. Guaranteed.
Ships Federal Express Next Day to ensure freshness.*

The Sproutpeople's Organic Sprout Wonderland
225 Main St
Gays Mills, WI 54631
Tel (877) -SPROUTS
http://www.sproutpeople.com

Nature's Path Foods, Inc.
7453 Progress Way
Delta, BC, Canada
V4G 1E8
Tel (604) 940-0505
http://www.naturespath.com
Offers sprouted manna bread

Omega Nutrition USA
6515 Aldrich Road
Bellingham, WA 98226
Tel. (360) 384-1238
Fax (360) 384-0700
http://www.omeganutrition.com
High quality oils

Air Cleaners

AllerMed Corporation
312 Steel Road
Wylie, TX 75098
Tel (978) 442-4898
http://www.allermedcleanair.com

Allerx Air Cleaners
PO Box 1119
Royse City, TX 75189
Tel (972) 635-2580
Fax (800) 929-9712
http://www.allerx.com

EL Foust Co
PO BOX 105
Elmhurst, IL. 60126
Tel (800) EL-FOUST
Fax (630) 834-5341
http://www.foustco.com

Alpine Air Purifiers
Tel (316) 686-1793
Fax (316) 685-5301
http://www.alpine-air-purifiers-usa.com

Water Purifiers

American Environmental Health Foundation
8345 Walnut Hill Lane, Suite 225
Dallas, TX 75231
Tel (214) 361-9515
http://www.aehf.com

Sun-Pure
5407 E. La Palma Avenue
Anaheim, California 92807
Tel (714) 779-2220
Fax (714) 779-8277
http://www.sun-pure.com

Non-Toxic Home Improvement Supplies

American Environmental Health Foundation
8345 Walnut Hill Lane, Suite 225
Dallas, TX 75231
Tel (214) 361-9515
http://www.aehf.com

Saunas

Sauna Store
P.O. Box 3722
Cherry Hill, NJ 08034
Tel (856) 489-1594
Fax (856) 489-1106
http://www.saunastore.com

Northernlight Saunas
167 Clinton Ave.
Kingston, NY 12401
Tel (800) 344-0513
Fax (914) 340-1732
http://www.northernlightsaunas.com

APPENDIX H

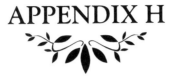

Naturopathic Physician's Oath

Naturopathic Physician's Oath

I dedicate myself to the service of humanity
as a practitioner of the art and science of Naturopathic medicine.

I will honor my teachers and all
who have preserved and developed this knowledge
and dedicate myself to supporting the growth and evolution of Naturopathic medicine.
I will endeavor to continually improve my abilities
as a healer through study, reflection and genuine concern for humanity.
I will impart knowledge of the advanced healing arts
to dedicated colleagues and students.

Through precept, lecture and example,
I will assist and encourage others to strengthen their health,
reduce risks for disease and preserve the health of our planet
for ourselves, our families and future generations.

According to my best ability and judgment,
I will use methods of treatment
which follow the principles of Naturopathic medicine :

First of all, to do no harm.

To act in cooperation with the Healing Power of Nature.

To address the fundamental causes of disease.

To heal the whole person through individualized treatment.

To teach the principles of healthy living and preventive medicine.

I will conduct my life and the practice of Naturopathic health care
with vigilance, integrity and freedom from prejudice.
I will abstain from voluntary acts of injustice and corruption.
I will keep confidential whatever I am privileged to witness,
whether professionally or privately, that should not be divulged.

With my whole heart, before this gathering of witnesses
as a
Doctor of Naturopathic Medicine
I pledge to remain true to this oath.

INDEX

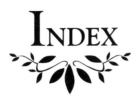

D – F

G – I

J – L

M – O

P – R

ABOUT THE AUTHOR

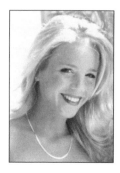

Gina L. Nick, Ph.D., N.D. is a Doctor of Naturopathic Medicine and a recognized Researcher in the area of Nutritional Science. She is a graduate of Southwest College of Naturopathic Medicine and Health Sciences and the University of California, Los Angeles. She graduated from UCLA with Latin and College honors and received distinguished honors from SCNM for her work in nutritional biochemistry, microbiology, homeopathy and botanical medicine. She is Vice President of Research and Development at Longevity Through Prevention, Inc., a health consulting firm. Her expertise in nutritional medicine has earned her awards and grants to study in the United States and abroad. As a researcher, she identified and devised a method for measuring the effectiveness of nutritional formulations intracellularly on live cells using a chemiluminescent dye and molecular probe, and has a patent pending on her process (Optical Antioxidant Sensing Process™). She is also the researcher and formulator of a variety of highly reputable nutritional supplements that have been proven clinically effective through experimental in-vitro as well as clinical in-vivo research studies. She is the author of numerous published and peer-reviewed scientific documents that focus on validating the use of key nutrient combinations, primarily as they naturally occur in whole foods and herbs. She is a member of the UCLA Alumni Scholar Association, the American Association of Naturopathic Physicians, the American Medical Writers Association, the American Nutraceutical Association and the American Holistic Health Association. Dr. Nick's clinical experience as a Naturopathic Physician, coupled with her findings as a researcher, reinforced her passion to communicate to every health care practitioner the need to have a comprehensive understanding of the Clinical Purification™ process if one's intent is to assist the body in healing itself from disease.

Contact Information:

Gina L. Nick, Ph.D., N.D.
PO Box 627
Brookfield, WI 53008
drgina@ltponline.com